A Better Way To Marry:

A Family Approach To Lasting Love For Generations

Ken and Verena Hardman

Book cover designer is Donna Harriman Murillo.

DEDICATION

We dedicate this book to our parents for their unconditional love, to our children and to future generations.

TABLE OF CONTENTS

ACKNOWLEDGMENTS

We are grateful to those who have encouraged us during the past 14 years while researching and writing this book— caring parents and their adult children who desire to get marriage right from the start. We also have been motivated by the dedication and needs of parents whose public service in the nonprofit and government foreign service, and in military and religious organizations, has incurred additional burdens on their marriages and families.

Thank you Josie Hauer for introducing us to a wide range of marriage and family educators who continue to enlighten us with their research: educators like John M. Gottman, Stephen R. Covey, John Gray, Martin E. P. Seligman, Gary D. Chapman, Les Parrott III and Leslie Parrott, James E. Hughes Jr., John Van Epp and many more.

Special thanks to Mose Durst, our friend and scholar whose reminders to write simply and clearly have led to this book's current form. As Chairman of The Principled Academy, he and its staff and teachers have nurtured the heart and character of our children in K thru 8th grade. Their commitment to character education, parent involvement, and the daily practice of virtues provides us with lessons for marriage readiness and family development.

Other friends and colleagues have shared with us encouragement and advice: Bento Leal, a humorful and masterful instructor of marriage and family communication skills; Don Sardella, an experienced and compassionate business consultant whose astute insights have advanced our understanding how both careers and families can be enriched. There are more and we apologize for not mentioning them all.

We thank our daughter Jeanina who, with her keen eye, has added another layer of editing to this book.

Thank you and hugs to all our children who have trusted us and share with us a commitment to the vision of generations of healthy, happy marriages and families.

PREFACE

Where did the romantic belief come from that falling in love leads to happiness and should be the basis for marriage?

This may be a question you never thought about. Although love is a *many-splendored thing*, it is difficult for most people to talk about love and what it is.

Why do people repeatedly fall in and out of love? Have you ever asked, "How can some-*thing* feel so good yet turn out so bad?"

If people know that romantic love is blind and there is such *a thing* as love sickness, why do they want to experience that *thing*?

Why do many therapists think that the unstable mental state of falling in love—the *thing*--is a legitimate precondition and basis for marriage? Why are so many of them inclined to think that parents don't know how to guide their children when it comes to marriage, even though parents have the legal duty to socialize their children to become responsible adults?

Have you ever wondered why parents have a hard time talking with their children about marriage? When their son or daughter experiences an intense romantic attraction, a "thing," how do parents help them to safely and wisely determine whether their object of desire has the potential to be a good, reliable, lifelong mate, to be a good "match?"

Have you ever lamented, "There must be a better way for single adults to marry, other than by 'following their heart' through the risky dating scene where dishonesty is common, hearts are broken, and sexual assault is widespread?"

Have you ever wondered whether there is a way to marry that better assures a couple gets marriage right from the start?

These are the kinds of questions that we will be addressing in this book.

Why Read This Book?

A Better Way To Marry provides tools for evaluating marriage readiness. These tools are helpful for anyone seeking an informed and meaningful basis for choosing a marital partner and forming a healthy marriage. *A Better Way To Marry* enables a broader perspective for meaningful reflection and conversation about lasting love, romance, intimacy and sexuality in marriage. It teaches how to form a marriage as part of a supportive network of families.

Who Can Benefit from This Book?

- Anyone seeking a safe, wise, and reliable basis for choosing a lifelong partner and forming a happy, fulfilling marriage. *A Better Way To Marry* provides concepts and a vocabulary to understand and talk about love, intimacy and marriage, and explains what to look for in a potential marriage partner.

- Singles tired of the disappointments, dishonesty, hazards and heartbreaks in the contemporary dating scene. While we encourage single adults to partner with their parents to choose their life partner for marriage, even if they are unable to do so, this book provides helpful guidelines for self-matching or partnering with other trusted supporters.

- Parents (married or divorced) desiring to support their children to form healthy, happy marriages. They need not have had a perfect marriage to wisely coach their children to make the most important decision of their lives. We can all learn how to improve our levels of marital satisfaction and support one another to make our lives better together. Lifelong learning is for everyone.

- Parents who desire to heal strained relationships with their single adult children. Partnering with them to follow a safe and wise path to marriage can be a trust-building experience.

- Married couples seeking to enrich and enhance their marriages. The entry-level attitudes and relationship skills necessary to begin marriage are essential throughout a marriage. When parents mentor their children, they enrich their own marriage and demonstrate dedication to improve their marriage and be the best example that they can be for their children.

- Families desiring a sustainable basis for expanding intergenerational unity.

- High net-worth families concerned with risk management and wealth preservation. Family discord and nasty divorces can disrupt family businesses and bankrupt human and financial assets.

- Westerners desiring a more rational, success-formula approach to marriage.

- Those from Eastern cultures who hope to counter the trend of rising divorces among their children, and who value respect for elders, kinship, and family traditions.

What Is the Main Idea Here?

There is *A Better Way To Marry* that enables single adults to be better prepared for marriage, and, combined with their parents' and families' support, make decisions to marry that are better informed and meaningful, and that result in high levels of marital satisfaction and longevity. It is a better way than historically recent methods of premising marriage on risky dating and a short-lived, illusory mental state of romantic love, which has proven to be an unstable and unreliable basis for marriage.

A Better Way To Marry supports parents' labor of love to prepare their children for marriage. Providing parents with educational tools is a better way than presuming that they are incompetent when it comes to guiding their children to form a healthy marriage.

Let's look at the bigger picture. A healthy marriage is about maintaining healthy human relationships. Finding and forming a marriage with a Mr. or Ms. Right is first about being a Mr. or Ms. Right--a healthy human being who can form and sustain healthy relationships, especially in marriage.

Unfortunately, America's cultural deck of cards is stacked against getting marriage right from the start.

Waiting Till It Is Too Late

People seek relationship education usually after it is too late (nearly 50% of couples divorce). It is called "couple's therapy," sought after suffering for 1, 5, 10, 20 or more years of marriage. When it comes to marriage, the other place that people seek relationship education and training is "pre-marriage counseling." However, that can be too late as well. Why? Because a couple is usually happy with one another at that time, and they have already made up their minds to marry—they are engaged. What if, though, without realizing it, they picked the wrong person for a mate? One or both may have deep-seated negative habits, lack healthy relationship skills and be unprepared for marriage.

How about those who don't seek out relationship education and training? In America, marriage preparedness is more associated with a checklist of action items for a big, blowout wedding. It is far less connected with the attitudes, skills and habits necessary to begin and maintain a healthy marriage and family. Pre-marriage relationship education is often dismissed by singles who regard themselves as a "couple" and who argue that they don't need it since they are not yet married. What happens after they marry? They often just as quickly dismiss marriage education as something only for couples in crisis.

Entry-Level Readiness Is Required

Yes, people often wait till it is too late to seek relationship education and training to prepare themselves for marriage. Becoming an *adult* is a transformational process that requires time, knowledge and stepping stone experiences to apply that knowledge. Like beginning a new job, having matured to be a responsible adult is an entry-level prerequisite to begin the transformational process of *becoming* a healthy, responsible, caring *husband or wife*. Similarly, "becoming" a healthy, capable *parent* is also a transformational process and entry-level readiness is required.

The best time for relationship education and training is before you enter into marriage, well before you are engaged, and well before thinking about marrying a particular person. Preparing for marriage is like preparing for a career: education and training are necessary to develop entry-level readiness and competencies. Preparing for marriage is about becoming a healthy adult, able to develop healthy relationships, which can be called romantic competence.

However, who are the best people to teach and where is the best place to learn how to become a healthy, responsible adult, able to form healthy, responsible relationships in marriage and in a family? How about in one's family of origin and from one's parents? But where and from whom do parents learn how to socialize their children to become healthy adults prepared for marriage and parenting? You can walk that question back to each previous generation. We learn from those who came before us.

At the same time, a perfect storm of historical and cultural changes has negatively impacted anyone seeking to get marriage right from the start. The storm has resulted in the loss of a coherent framework to talk about love, in "generation gaps" that impair family unity and parents' ability to socialize their children for marriage, and the ability of single adults to form and maintain a healthy marriage.

Confused Rites of Passage into Adulthood

Consider contemporary culture in America. It has lost its rites of passage that define when boys become men and girls become women. Adolescence is prolonged and many boys think that a defining act of passage is having sex; some join violent gangs as alternative families, where manhood is defined by robbing or killing.

The pervasive influences of pop culture promote false images of what it means to be a man and a woman. Both men and women are objectified. Unrealistic images of the perfect body lead girls to seek ultra-thinness, often causing anorexia and bulimia, and lead boys to use steroids, in the hope of becoming super muscular and powerful in sports. The images may lead them to live under a cloud of self-declared inadequacy and belittled self-worth. While seeking love and acceptance in all the wrong places, the false images may lead them into risky behaviors and toxic relationships.

In our postmodern age of equality, the culture-wide ethical ideal for male-female relationships—a gentleman and lady—has been discarded without a replacement. As a consequence, virtues such as heroism, honor, humility and modesty have been marginalized. Male and female relations are more confused than ever and have been reduced to debates over dominance and a not-so-funny struggle for power, the battle of the sexes.

Self-Esteem and Romantic Love Have Replaced Character as Basis of Marriage

Joseph Campbell, a scholar of mythology, laments that Western religions are "out of sync" with contemporary society, and are not applying their teachings in today's world. That results in young people disengaging from the wisdom of religions' spiritual messages. Singles are left alone to create their own meanings about male-female relationships and marriage in a culture that stresses individualism, immediate gratification, materialism, and technology, a culture which reduces equality to sameness.[1]

The idea of self-esteem has replaced a societal standard of honorable, moral behavior. An individual's self-esteem can fluctuate like a gas gauge, depending on how they perceive acceptance or rejection from others. Like the gauge of self-esteem, the feelings of romantic love can also swing radically from full to empty. Self-esteem and romantic love have within our Western culture replaced the wisdom and virtues of the world's great religions as the basis of marriage. Contemporary marriage has become fragile and its stature as a sacred institution has been reduced to just another piece of paper, another transaction and option in life.

Contemporary Dating Is Not Safe or Smart
Dating Replaced Courtship

One reason that marriages today are fragile, often fail, or are compromised before they begin, is that dating is disconnected from marriage. From the 1880s through the 1920s, dating gradually replaced "calling" as the form of courtship, a formal process through which a man and a woman explored the possibilities of becoming married.

Dating Is Disconnected from Marriage

As marriage became more optional, the purpose of dating was no longer exclusively courtship for marriage.

Today the purpose of dating is generally focused on pleasure, having fun, enhancing self-esteem, and being emotionally and physically gratified without commitment. Dating is often the search for "The One," "The Perfect One."

Dating Is Approached Like Shopping

Have you heard the lament "Where did all the good ones go?" The reasons given for a *Mr. or Miss Not Good Enough* are endless: he is not romantic enough, exciting enough, attractive enough, energetic enough; he is too short, too boring, too bald, too cheerful; her body is not "hot" enough. The thinking is "I'm not settling for anything less." Dating is approached like shopping: There are endless fish in the sea and they are within the reach of your fingertips, from online sites such as Tinder, OKCupid, to Sonar. Friends ask, "How would you rate your date on a scale of 1 to 10?" A reply might be that "he/she is a 7 or 8, but not a knock-your-socks-off 9 or 10."

Hooking Up Is Trending to Replace Dating

Sociologist Kathleen A. Bogle explains that over the past 60 years, traditional forms of courting and dating have been replaced by "hooking up", that is casual, uncommitted sexual encounters between people who are not dating or romantically involved. Hooking up has become common among adolescents, emerging adults, and men and women in Western culture. On college campuses hooking up has become the normative way heterosexual students get together.[2]

Dating Is Not Safe--Violence Is Common

Considering the physical and emotional risks of contemporary dating, it is like Russian roulette. The Centers for Disease Control (CDC) report that dating violence in the United States is a serious problem which regularly occurs: "1 in 5 high school girls has been physically or sexually abused by a dating partner....54% of students report dating violence among their peers."[3]

A new trend called "stealthing," the non-consensual removal of a condom before or during sex, is reported by Alexandra Brodsky in the *Columbia Journal of Gender and Law*. She explains that its male proponents justify it by belief in male supremacy and dominance. The practice can threaten "to destroy the normalcy of dating, or 'hooking up'".[4]

Online Dating Websites: Can You Tell the Truth?

In our brave new world, singles are placing their trust in technology to find their soulmate. Savvy marketers declare that their online dating systems with special algorithms provide a "scientific" approach to matchmaking, even a "secret sauce." New matchmaking intermediaries offer their services as relationship professionals, dating coaches and matchmakers, who themselves may not have a healthy marriage. Their strategy appeals as business concepts of outsourcing to experts and an overriding trust in science and technology. They have replaced the traditional advisory and intermediary roles of parents, family, and religious leaders. Unfortunately, online dating website profiles are notoriously filled with distortions and lies.[5]

Contemporary Dating:
Inadequate Foundation for Marriage

Contemporary dating lacks structure and rituals that prepare and connect individuals to the realities of marriage and the wisdom of life. As hooking up and dating are centered on self-gratification and romantic love is glorified, singles enter into a "relationship" or marriage…blind. With the focus on experiencing the euphoric emotions of falling in love, the fog, intensity and unrealistic expectations of romantic love can impede genuine discovery and real understanding. When people date, they are not inclined to think or ask about the realities of marriage: "How would it be building a life together with this person? Having children? Dealing with life's joys, sickness, disappointments, unemployment? Growing old together?" Marriage requires a shift in one's personal identity from "me" to "we." Left alone, singles may not realize and genuinely commit to the greater transcendent good of "we."

Couples often enter marriage without discussing the foundational issues of marriage. That sets them up for disappointment, as they skate into their new life together, thinking that they can sustain a long-term relationship on the feelings of chemistry and fireworks.

If married couples have poor communication skills, they may emotionally "drift apart," engage in criticizing one another's character and personality, and express contempt, defensiveness and stonewalling.[6] When couples inevitably fall out of the illusory in-love state, it is easy to feel that dreams were betrayed. Many choose to divorce, or they may endure an unhappy marriage; or hopefully, when the illusions of romantic love have evaporated, they recommit to renewal and learn how to love in a genuine, skillful and enduring manner.

Why do so many people overlook issues and warning signs in their dating relationships and continue to have the same problems afflict their marriages years later? Romantic love is blind and intoxicating. Have you ever heard a friend recovering from a divorce or broken relationship lament, "If only I knew then what I know now"?

Again, who are the best persons to teach and mentor singles to become prepared for marriage? How about their parents and other elders? While some people agree, others may not. Let us consider why that could be.

Presumed Parental Incompetence

During the past century, a growing societal presumption emerged that marriage should be privatized, that parents should keep their distance and not be involved in their children's selection of a spouse or in their marriages.

In traditional societies around the world and at the turn of the twentieth century in America, younger members of a family and community were mentored by elders—parents, aunts and uncles—to assume the role of adults, to marry and be parents.

Since the turn of the twentieth century, when young people migrated from rural areas to big cities, psychiatrists, psychologists and marriage counselors--newly formed and unproven professions--gradually replaced traditional social support systems formerly provided by parents, elders, priests, pastors, and rabbis. Even though there has been no serious scientific study of love, marriage, and happiness until the past 40 years, Sigmund Freud's complex, fatalistic, sex-based theories of love, human nature and psychoanalysis were unquestioned through most of the twentieth century and accepted as dogma...like a religion.[7] Freud and his intellectual heirs declared that a child's relationship to his parent, especially the mother, was responsible for everything from insomnia, impotence, to psychiatric disorders and criminal behavior. The parent was to blame. Educator Laurence Peter joked, "Psychiatry enables us to correct our faults by confessing our parents' shortcomings."[8]

Mental health professions, still in their formative stages and internally divided, have in broad strokes blamed parents and discouraged them from believing that they can trust themselves to learn how to raise their children to become healthy adults and that they know more than they think they do. Parental incompetence is often presumed. Ask any one of them if they think parents can adequately prepare their children for marriage.

Consider, as a practical matter, that a large percentage of mental health practitioners and academics are probably parents. They, their marriages and their families are not exempt from addictions, depression, mental disorders and family discord, nor do they always take their own advice.

The Fix?

So, what is the fix for inadequate preparation for marriage and parenting? More of the same? The normative vision of marriage for the majority of Americans is for two singles to date, experience chemistry, fall in love and marry (maybe); and, of course, their parents should not be involved. How well does that work?

Tweens, teens and young adults are left to walk alone in the minefields of dating where violence is widespread. Violence continues in marriages and has reached epidemic proportions. Also, about 50% of first marriages end in divorce and the percentages increase with each remarriage. Divorce is the new normal and is regarded as acceptable. If autos or bridges had the same failure rate, would the public accept that and their faulty designs?

So, what is the fix? Rely upon technology through online dating and algorithms—more accurately called online "introductions" --to choose one's mate? Rely on the mythologies of romantic love to guide you to "the Perfect One"? Presume that parents should keep their noses out of their children's dating and choice of a spouse? That there is a red line to their involvement?

Enable Parents
To Be Wisdom Givers for Marriage

It is time to exercise some common sense and collaboration to support the position of parents and help one another's families learn the skills to become healthy adults. We all have difficulty dealing with our imperfections. The lack of culture-wide models of virtuous men and women, a healthy marriage, and the presumed incompetence of parents do not help. It is time for our society to face reality and recognize the responsibility, capacity, and benefits of parents to socialize their children for marriage from a platform that does not perpetuate cycles of abuse and divorce.

The notion of presumed parental incompetence contradicts the fiduciary responsibility of parents owed their children, the highest level of care, loyalty and good faith imposed by our legal system. Parents are required to act in their children's best interests to raise them to become responsible adults both in public and in private.

Socialization is the process of inheriting and transferring ideals to the next generation: values, virtues, a normative vision, system of beliefs and worldview that explain a society's acceptable ways to believe and act in public and private. Socialization is educating the next generation with skills and habits necessary to live by those ideals as responsible adults in society. Socialization is the way a society sustains and perpetuates itself.

Parents Should and Can Become the Experts

Are parents supposed to be perfect and make no mistakes? We are all the fruit of the past. We can all make new beginnings. Whether as a husband, wife, father, mother, son or daughter, brother or sister, growing in love is about humility, forgiving, healing and making new beginnings.

Being a spouse and a parent is a discipline. Parents teach by their example. With a little coaching they can identify and surface their learned wisdom about marriage, to explain, refine, and confidently teach it to their children. That is what marriage and family researchers do like John Gottman in his couples' "Love Lab"[9]: they search for and distill that inner wisdom of husbands and wives, fathers and mothers, which are identified as best practices. Parents can be and should be the marriage experts in their family, and not presume that they must "outsource to other experts" their parental responsibilities to prepare for and partner with their children to form their marriages.

Marriage and Parenting Are Learnable Skills

A Better Way To Marry provides tools, coherent concepts, a working vocabulary, and prudent practices to support parents and single adults to get marriage right from the start.

Recognizing that the social sciences are in their formative stages and often internally divided, the recommended ideas and processes in this book are based on their commonalities and points of research agreement in the studies of human, marriage and family development, Western romantic love marriages and Eastern arranged marriages.

Marriage is a spiritual discipline that requires lifelong learning about lasting love, romance and intimacy. Parenting is also a spiritual discipline in which we are challenged to pass the best of the past to next generations.

Today, it is more important than ever for single adults who desire to marry to collaborate closely with their families. Millions of families in the US were overwhelmed by the financial meltdown of the Great Recession and foreclosure evictions. Hurricane Sandy also brought havoc to millions of families on the East Coast. A Pew Research Center study reported that in the past decade, 24% of young adults 18 to 34 have remained or have moved back in with their parents or parents-in-law.[10] That is more than 24 million. There is also "data showing that nearly 60 percent of 23- to 25-year-olds report receiving some kind of financial assistance from their parents."[11] American notions of rugged individualism and self-reliance are romanticized. Yes, like romantic love, those beliefs are exaggerated, glorified and unrealistic.

A New Approach to Marriage Is Needed

A new framework for conversation and cooperation between the generations is required. The adversarial mindset of generational conflicts will not solve the problems of the present or the future. It will make them worse. Indeed, a cooperative mindset is far better. Forming new marriages that become strong links in the chain of families provide opportunities to be better together.

We introduce you to *A Family Approach To Lasting Love For Generations*. It includes a flexible framework for informed conversation and cooperation between the generations. Since preparing for and choosing a life partner for marriage is about predicting a person's potential and future behavior as a spouse, a parent, and an in-law, we walk you through a discussion of human nature, character and personality, healthy relationships, sexuality, marriage and family. They form the basis for realistic expectations for a healthy human being that are prerequisites for marriage. These prerequisites are condensed within Three Benchmarks for basic marriage readiness and their predictive Indicators.

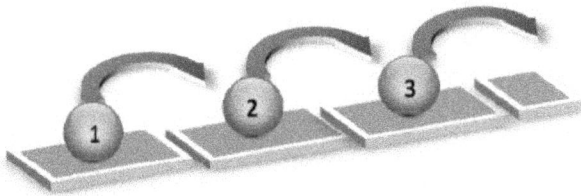

This flexible framework guides parents and their single adult sons and daughters through a layered, reflective discovery process of writing and discussion that builds trust, self-knowledge and mutual understanding, and also serves as a common yardstick to evaluate potential marital candidates. Learning about oneself and others is about asking and answering meaningful questions. More than 200 Indicator questions and their meanings are provided from which to select as needed. Remember, there is no need to use them all.

CHAPTER 1:
WITH THE END IN MIND

"We may not be able to prepare the future for our children, but we can at least prepare our children for the future." - President Franklin D. Roosevelt

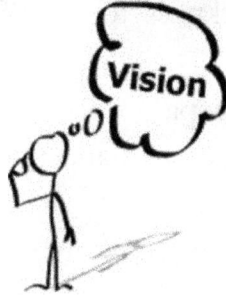

A Better Way To Marry has a clear end in mind: a vision of healthy marriages and families. You can create that vision, personalized for you, and a strategy that pulls your family together for generations.

Needed Paradigm Shifts

Considering the heartbreaking track record of broken contemporary marriages, *A Better Way To Marry* involves some paradigm shifts necessary to form healthy relationships and marriages. They encompass common myths, stereotypes and misconceptions about male-female relationships, love, romance, intimacy, marriage and family:

- From marriage as an afterthought to marriage as a forethought,
- From unrealistic to realistic expectations about marriage,
- From falling in love to growing in love; from love just happens to love is learned,

1

- From false/illusory romance to true/genuine romance,
- From false/illusory chemistry to true/genuine chemistry,
- From love sickness to love fitness; from pathology to well-being,
- From a prepackaged-in-heaven soulmate to becoming a soulmate and nurturing the soul of your mate,
- From waiting for the "only One" in the universe to "becoming as one,"
- From self-centered purpose to transcendent purpose,
- From a hormonal high as the basis of marriage to character readiness as the basis of marriage,
- From dishonest profiles to honest profiles,
- From disrespectful communication to respectful communication,
- From surviving to thriving in marriage,
- From uncertain and temporary intimacy to reliable and sustained intimacy,
- From dependent and independent marriages and families to interdependent marriages and families,
- From one generation to seven-generational thinking.

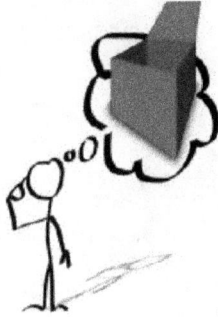

3 Big Ideas

Those paradigm shifts involve safer, more effective human technologies and three big ideas:

1. Positive generation thinking and kinship building,
2. Being prepared for marriage, and
3. Using a safe and smart marriage-formation process.

Big Idea # 1

Positive Generation Thinking & Kinship Building

Thinking in terms of generations is not a new idea. However, since the 1960s, relationships between generations are commonly thought of in negative terms, such as generation gaps. Communication and cooperation between young people and their parents and grandparents are regarded as difficult. Such gaps existed before the 1960s, though.[12]

Strained communication is not the only problem. There is also the historical pattern of family wealth lost over three generations, which is observed in many cultures and known as the "rags-to-riches-to-rags" cycle, or "rags-to-rags in three generations" where both the second and third generation squander the wealth of the first generation.[13]

Therefore, a positive end in mind is needed that envisions generations of families preserving and *transferring the best of life beyond three generations.*

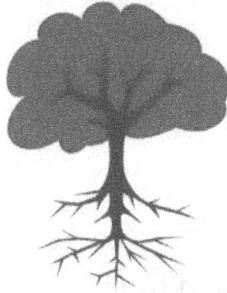

Cultivating the Family Tree

Consider the metaphor of planting and cultivating a copper beech tree, which sixth-generation counselor-at-law James E. Hughes Jr. likens to the generational thinking and practices needed to develop a "compact among generations." A copper beech tree grows to maturity in about 150 years. When a gardener plants this tree, he trusts that if it is planted and maintained properly, it can root and sprout. If the trunk can get a good start by growing straight for a few years, it is likely to grow to maturity. Similarly, a clear vision and guiding principles are essential to develop strong and healthy families for generations.[14]

Paradigm shifts--fundamental changes in one's assumptions or approach--are not easy to make. Thinking in terms of many future generations, not just one or two generations, but seven, is a challenge. Some families, though, have stuck together through thick and thin for many generations. Such families provide models for how it can be done. They include, not surprisingly, a shared vision, a family code of conduct, an infrastructure of elders, and a tradition of values, virtues and principles that each new generation buys into.

Wealthy parents are concerned about teaching and guiding their children to preserve wealth. Many were seriously shaken by the global stock market meltdown of the Great Recession, which caused them to question the basis of how they do business and with greater consideration for their children's future.[15] Most would hope their children will succeed under any economic circumstance. For that to happen, though, more is involved than sensible spending and saving patterns. It involves helping children define success, the nature of wealth, and to discover their life purposes and define their priorities.

An Equal Opportunity Approach

Lower and middle-class parents similarly hope the best for their families. Rethinking wealth and family relationships will help to restore the American Dream. Planning and collaborating over many generations can better assure equal opportunity for future generations to live dignified and meaningful lives.

Generation Thinking to the Past: Family History

A positive end in mind includes understanding the past because it shapes the present and can influence the future for good or ill. Each person is a "work in progress," and for better or worse, brings their past into a marriage. Sometimes habits from the past, like software, have flaws and need to be repaired.

When committing yourself to another person for the rest of your life, it is essential to know the inner life of your mate and who and what has shaped their character. Genetic and family behavioral traits may have been repeated for generations in the family lineage. Family history can reveal strengths and weaknesses of a potential mate. It is important to be aware how a potential mate's family interacted.

To the Future: Strategic Planning

A positive end in mind for a family is about loving and caring kinship. It is a vision of people related by birth and marriage, nurturing and supporting one another to be healthy, happy and prosperous. When that is put in writing, it becomes a family vision statement.

In your family vision statement, visualize many generations of healthy, happy, prosperous marriages and families that support and nurture one another. It can be a leap of faith for some people to do that, especially when their sense of connectedness with generations only extends back to a few memories of grandparents.

Let a hopeful vision be a part of your end in mind. Let it not only help you and your children form healthy marriages, but also lay the groundwork for later extended family development.

Serious generation thinking and kinship building involve strategic planning, which presumes that you can shape your future by taking action today. Step forward with that belief, and identify stepping-stone action items like the following:

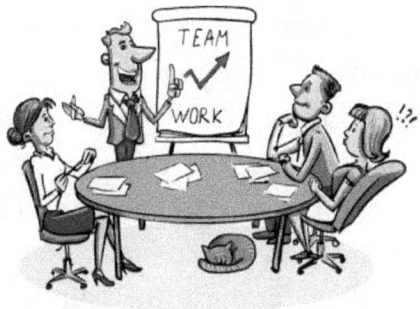

- Develop marriage and family literacy. Educate yourselves and your children with the best literature and research about healthy marriages and families.
- Guide your children to develop transferable social skills needed in a healthy marriage.
- Develop benchmarks and indicators to assess and predict whether your unmarried children and potential mates are ready for marriage, compatible and complementary.
- Develop trust and confidence in your family's ability to collaborate and make new beginnings.
- Enable your children to make informed, meaningful decisions in their choice of a lifelong mate and to form healthy, happy, prosperous marriages.
- Encourage a vision and commitment for continued interdependent collaboration among your married children and the families of their spouses.

These action items are like design features in a suspension bridge that can join and sustain two families through marriage into the distant future.

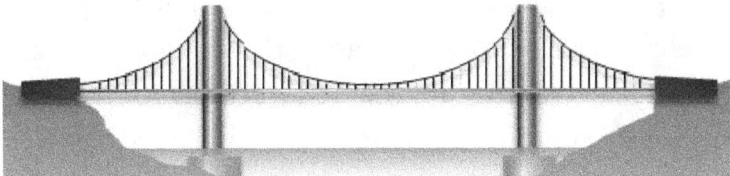

Big Idea #2: Marital Readiness

The second big idea is for single adults to be ready for marriage. Sounds too simple, doesn't it? Marriage should be a forethought and not an afterthought. Readiness is about being a healthy adult who understands what marriage is about and is prepared for it.

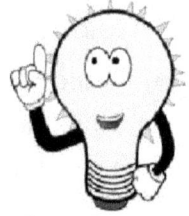

When emotional discipline and relationship skills are lacking, destructive habits and unrealistic expectations can be formed, which heighten the potential for conflict and neglect or abuse.

If single adults have basic readiness for marriage, they can adjust and *grow* through the various stages of marriage to expand their scope of responsible caring as husbands and wives and as fathers and mothers.

Roles may be reversed as couples get older. Men often initially prioritize their careers above intimacy in their marriage, but reverse that when they hit a career ceiling or become unemployed or unable to work. During that reversal of a man's priorities, women may seek fulfillment through a vocation just when their husbands are giving more attention to their marriages.

A prudent approach to marriage is not to expect to find a flawless soulmate. Don't base your marriage expectations on an elitist, perfectionistic standard. No one is a finished product when entering marriage. Every person brings into marriage a unique personality with strengths and weaknesses. A couple's combination of strengths and weaknesses produces issues that must be acknowledged and managed.

Be Basically Healthy

When entering into marriage, expect yourself and your children and their mates to be basically healthy-- emotionally, mentally, spiritually and socially.

Marriages that end in divorce, even after 10 or 20 years, usually were in trouble before they began. They survived– for a time–but did not thrive. Engaged couples tend to avoid relationship issues and spend more time preparing for their wedding than for their marriage. The euphoria of being in love easily obscures their sense of reality.

Within the context of romantic love marriages, it is less common for men and women to think that they must prove themselves worthy and prepared to be someone's spouse. The typical presumption is that one is qualified to marry if one experiences the euphoria of "being in love." Singles, thinking that they are being humble, might say, "I won't know if I'm ready for marriage until I fall in love with 'the One.' Only love knows." Asserting unquestionable independence, the expectation for marriage fitness could rally a call of indignation, "Who are you to judge me? I am an individual, an adult!"

Asking the Right Questions

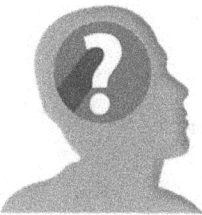

Ask good questions and wisely evaluate the answers. Beyond a few generalities, typically people do not know what questions to ask regarding marriage readiness. Try asking this question to single adults hoping to marry/or to parents of single adults hoping to marry:

9

- Why do you think you are ready for marriage?
- Why do you think your son/daughter is ready for marriage?

There will be a wide range of responses, but most will struggle with an answer. It is a difficult question. Some will be stunned by the question, and a few will acknowledge that they had not thought much about it.

People can become defensive when asked a question that they don't know how to answer. If you are a parent and were asked that question about your unmarried adult son or daughter, what would you reply? If you are single, what would you answer about yourself?

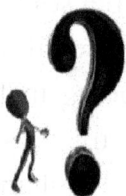

When college-educated singles desiring marriage are asked, "Are you ready for marriage?", common replies include, "No one is ever really ready," "I believe that I understand the level of commitment required," or simply, "I feel that I am ready."

Corporate hiring managers know that the content of questions, how and when they are asked, shape the applicants' answers and how well they are matched with a job description. Likewise, we all are challenged to ask meaningful questions about our most important human experiences. Ask *yourself*:

- Considering that a healthy marriage requires two healthy partners, what is a healthy human being?
- Related to that, what is entry-level readiness for marriage?
- What is love and true love fitness and how can these be measured?

- How do you measure compatibility and complementariness?
- What attitudes, skills and experiences are indications that a person can develop genuine intimacy, be a good team player in marriage and family, and unconditionally commit to marriage for a lifetime?

Big Idea # 3: A Safe, Smart, Marriage-Formation Process

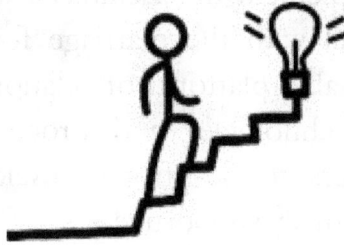

Aside from knowing how to assess whether you or your children and their potential mates are ready for marriage, it is another challenge to design an intentional marriage process that is safe, and guides all parties through simple steps of meaningful discovery and verification.

Two generations of the Roebling family led a team of engineers to construct the Brooklyn Bridge in the nineteenth century. Their determination, faith, personal sacrifices and teamwork enabled them to discover breakthroughs in technology that made it possible for the bridge to be built in 1883 and to become one of the oldest suspension bridges in the United States. The collaboration of those two generations and their new technologies were critical for the bridge to become safe and sustainable for current and future generations. Similarly, breakthroughs in human technology and intergenerational unity are needed

11

to create the foundations and social infrastructures that can support marriages and families for many generations.

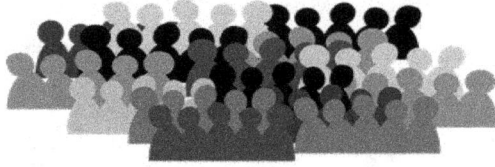

Civil engineers collaborate with architects. They use technologies and devise the structures and materials that support and complement the architect's vision and design. There is a parallel with the marriage formation process. Building a sustainable platform of relationships requires a vision, human technologies and processes that inspire individual members to be strong, resilient, and to pull together to be mutually supportive.

Intend that your process of forming a marriage be an opportunity to strengthen trust within your family, and to

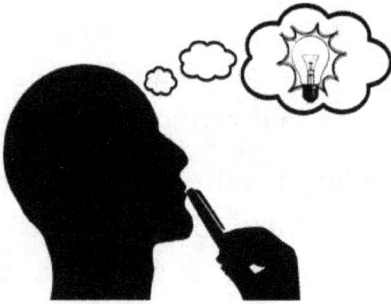

develop your collective decision-making skills. Unless you systematically develop your family-communication and decision-making skills to match your vision, the next generations can drift and fragment into isolated islands of busyness by default.

Ask yourselves:

- How can you reliably understand how and why a person's life is the way it is?
- How can you verify and be reasonably certain that answers from potential spouses are honest and revealing of who they are?

- How can you create an emotionally safe environment that enables meaningful discovery of yourself and potential spouses?
- What are the measures of a fully informed decision?
- How could you develop bridges for future collaboration with potential in-laws during the process?
- If you are a parent, how could you develop sustainable cooperation with your children, their spouses and in-laws and be a model for future generations?

Exploring whether someone could be a potential mate can be very emotional since one's feelings could be hurt in a variety of ways: There could be fear of rejection, of being judged (by others) as not good enough or getting stuck with the wrong one. Also, you may think that you are ready for marriage and have a clear idea of your ideal spouse, but later you realize that you are still confused about both.

Therefore, aim to create a safe environment with win-win outcomes that

- minimize fear,
- verify readiness for marriage, and
- provide opportunities for growth and self-discovery, even if no marriage were to result from discussions and courtship.

This book guides you through a process that can enable those outcomes.

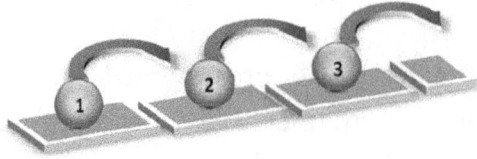

Slower is Better: Matchmaking is Slow Cooking

Slower is better because time is needed to genuinely discover whether someone is ready for marriage, compatible and complementary. Surprises and contradictions can surface. A meaningful choice requires full disclosure. If a single adult is to make a lifelong commitment to someone who will be their mutual helpmate, they need to know to whom they are committing and promising to help. When a person is accepted for both their strengths and weaknesses, trust is inspired and the attractive power of affection is stimulated.

A Better Way To Marry is about asking and answering good questions. It is about a slower, layered process that allows for the emergence of meaningful insights to gradually develop and be verified. It is like slow cooking.

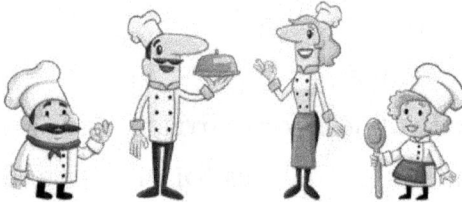

Slower is better to be sensitive and respectful to all the parties involved, to their personality types, hopes and dreams, stresses and uncertainties. Dialoguing with candidates and their parents is like learning to dance together. Thoughtful adjustments in the types, quantity and pacing of questions are made according to what is needed for genuine discovery.

A Layered Discovery Process

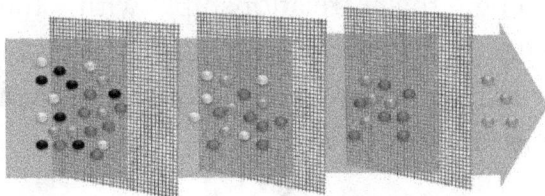

Discoveries in brain research reveal the brain's dual memory system. In one of the memories, buried within our unconscious, are correctly or incorrectly learned presumptions or mental models about how we should relate to ourselves, our families, others and the world around us. They are not repressed in the Freudian sense; we are simply not consciously aware of them. We intuitively sense them as feelings and are often unaware of how those presumptions affect our behavior unless we drill deep to discover the connections.

Cognitive linguist George Lakoff advises, "What people will tell you about their worldview does not necessarily accurately reflect how they reason, how they categorize, how they speak, and how they act."[16] Therefore, a layered approach to self-discovery and mutual discovery is essential to identify patterns of behaviors that predict readiness for marriage.

Although people are initially attracted by physical appearance, that is not what sustains a marriage. Part of a prudent, layered process is assessing your marital readiness—yours and that of a potential mate. This requires patience, honesty and humility with some coaching and mentoring.

Identify Parent-Child Issues

Evaluating a potential marriage partner includes understanding their relationship with their parents. Resentments and dysfunctional habits with one's parents can be carried into marriage and compromise relations with one's spouse and future in-laws.

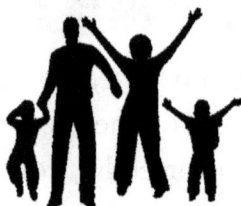

Don't be quick to jump to conclusions, though, about the candidate's parental relationship. As a society, we have been conditioned to believe that if the kids are good, the parents are good. If the kids are bad, the parents are bad. Such an over simplistic correlation is misleading.

It is true that the parents' personal examples, the way that they discipline, emotionally interact with and guide their children, influence their children's socialization—the way they think and act in everyday interactions with people. However, there are other influences in life, such as toxic popular culture messages and other derailing negative life experiences that lead a person to become involved in unhealthy relationships and make unhealthy life choices.

On the flip side, if a parent or parents are mentally troubled, that does not necessarily mean that their son or daughter is destined to be troubled. Therefore, it is necessary to take the time to understand a candidate's family history and not jump to conclusions.

If you are a parent, turn the mirror toward yourself, self-assess and do your best to assure that any resentments harbored by your children are resolved and that they and your relationship are healthy. No parent is "perfect." Any significant resentments or fears harbored by your children toward you could compromise their future marriages. They could also compromise your foundation of trust throughout the marriage formation process and into the future.

Identify Sibling Issues

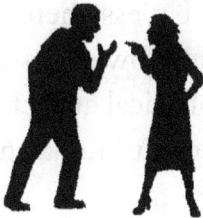

Sibling relationships can also have an important impact on how an individual behaves. This is a neglected area in developmental psychology. For good or ill, sibling squabbles teach kids how to negotiate and compromise, and how to tolerate negative emotions in a family. Siblings can learn positive or negative behaviors that are taken into adult life and marriage.

Children can be guided to follow family policies such as don't hurt one another; if you hurt your sibling, say, "I'm sorry," hug and give them a kiss; the sibling who was hurt says, "I forgive you." Do your best to instill within each child a sense that they are uniquely *special,* without the downsides of unrealistic entitlement. Feeling that you are genuinely loved and have been treated fairly in your family is basic to forming a healthy self-identity and minimizing the tendency to be jealous and resentful of others.

When single adults write their autobiographies and parents write biographies of their children desiring to marry, they benefit by sorting through and understanding their past family relationships and reasons for their views about love, marriage, parenting and family life. They also benefit those who are considering them as a potential mate or in-law.

Managing First Impressions

Another value of a well-thought-out, measured approach for selecting a lifelong marriage partner is to better manage the powerful first impressions of physical attraction, which can be very misleading. Unless there is a structured approach to marriage, which acknowledges and seriously considers factors in addition to physical attraction, two people who could otherwise become great life partners will not even consider one another.

A Family Approach

The three big ideas discussed in this chapter are part of a thoughtful, family approach to forming a marriage. Here is a basic outline of its seven steps:

- Step 1: Preparation (know thyself)
- Step 2: Identifying Candidates & Creating a Framework for Exploratory Discussions
- Step 3: Preliminary Fact-finding
- Step 4: Advanced Fact-finding
- Step 5: Pre-Courtship
- Step 6: Courtship to Pre-Engagement
- Step 7: Engagement and Pre-Marriage Preparation.

CHAPTER 2

STEP 1: PREPARATION-- BECOME STUDENTS OF MARRIAGE AND FAMILY

Science has only opened the doorway to understanding human nature. Its best role is not to be a pontificating high priest, but to be a servant that provides insights and tools for human well-being.

Arguably, the most important life decision that you or your children will make is whom to marry. The process of making that decision is not just about "finding" a Mr. Right or Ms. Right. It is also about first assuring that you are a Mr. Right or Ms. Right who is ready for marriage. What does it mean, though, to be ready for marriage? And how can anyone objectively determine this beyond romantic feelings, which can be very misleading, and beyond online website profiles, which can be very dishonest?

This chapter provides a flexible framework to think through these questions with a checklist of Three Benchmarks and predictive Indicators of marital readiness.

Become Lifelong Learners

There is widespread societal confusion about the nature of a healthy human being, love and marriage. You can be relieved to know that a man or woman need not be "fully formed" before marrying. After they marry, though, continued character development is required. Marital readiness is not about being "perfect." Put aside

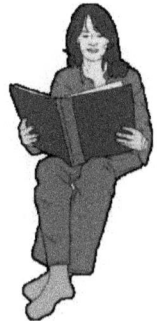

any fantasy belief you may have in soulmates who are pre-packaged in heaven.

When you dig deeper into existing research, you will discover that the social sciences are still in their infancy. Until the past 40 years, no serious scientific study of love, marriage and happiness was ever conducted, since as subjects they were considered not measurable. Also, the focus of psychology has been on pathology and not human well-being.

Social Sciences' Focus on Pathology and Theory

Commonly known as the founder of "Positive Psychology," Martin Seligman explains that at the end of WWII, the study of psychology in the universities had "nothing that was proven to work in the real world" and that would guide its research.[17] Academic focus has not been directed towards applied psychology needed for daily living; priority has been given to theoretical processes such as perception, cognition, and decision theory.

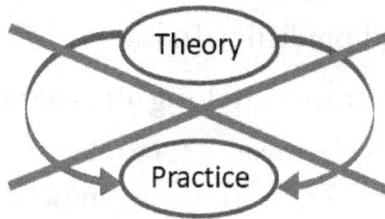

When Seligman was serving on a hiring committee at the University of Pennsylvania that was searching for a social psychologist in 1995, he discovered that not one tenured professor in the top 10 psychology departments in the world gave special attention to work, love or play. He asked, "Where were the scholars who would help guide us about what makes life worth living?"[18]

Pessimistic Theories of Human Nature

Freud's pessimistic theories of human nature has conjectured that love is rooted in sexual pleasure and perversion. His theories were widely accepted and unquestioned for most of the twentieth century. They were ineffective and, in many cases, counterproductive to healing the emotional problems of patients. Freud's doctrine of repressed memory buried in the unconscious mind included the presumption of incestuous thoughts for one's parents.

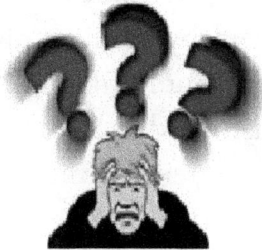

His repressed memory doctrine was stretched to include hiding purported gruesome memories of murder, which could be recovered through the assistance of a Freudian psychoanalyst. This theory was accepted as part of the expert opinion of psychiatrists in court trials.[19]

The doctrine of recovered repressed memory has since lost its credibility in the courts. In the 1990s, the effectiveness of pharmacology to treat depression, mood swings, anxiety, and delusions debunked Freud's doctrine of repressed sexual urges as the cause of emotional problems.[20]

Psychiatric medications have since become the dominant method of "fixing" mental illness. Sadly, though, medications have been overprescribed and have underperformed. The US does not have health care and mental health systems in primary care settings such as schools "that [are] accessible and adequately meet the needs of youth, adults and families." Therefore, mental health professionals have been pressured to provide expensive quick fixes with underperforming psychotropic medications. We have become an over-medicated society.[21]

Ordinary and Heroic Altruism Wrongly Denied

The study of human behavior in the twentieth century has focused on pathology and human sickness, and not on the measures of a healthy human being. Such an emphasis is mutually reinforced by fashionable evolutionary theory, which presumes that human beings are selfish by nature. Thus, acts of altruism and heroism are glibly dismissed as out of the ordinary pattern of human nature, even though they are performed by ordinary people.

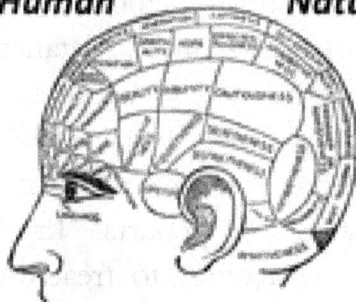

Heroism & Altruism Are Part Of Human Nature

New Research Dispels Myths

Longitudinal studies are emerging, which dispel long-held stereotypes and myths about adult, marriage and family development. Among them is psychiatrist George

Vaillant's Harvard Study of successful aging based on 72 years of interviews with those who have lived long and well.[22] Like psychologist Erik Erikson, Vaillant affirms that altruistic caring and giving to next generations, i.e., "generativity," is good for one's health. According to Vaillant, adult development is a new field of study and "still a mystery."[23] Long held theories about human nature and behavior have been disproved through new scientific discoveries in the past 20 years.

Seligman observed mental health illiteracy among over 90 percent of West Point cadets. While they had heard of post-traumatic stress disorder (PTSD), only 10% of them had heard of post-traumatic growth and resilience, which is a common experience. Seligman warns that such illiteracy can result in soldiers presuming that they have PTSD after a combat tragedy. This can aggravate normal grieving and tip soldiers over the edge into depression.[24]

Similarly, if couples presume that they must have a conflict-free marriage to be happy and with a continual euphoric high of romantic love, they may tragically conclude that they have a bad marriage and quickly look for the exit door when they feel emotionally stuck and unsatisfied.

Opening the Door

Neuroscience and pharmacology of the brain have opened the door to reexamining human nature, the nature of love and human relationships. Behavioral psychology and the doctrine of reward and punishment reigned supreme for many decades. John Watson, a famous behaviorist, warned against too much physical contact between mothers and their children because, as he argued, rewarding crying infants with attention would make them weak. John Bowlby's attachment theory that infants have an inborn need to be close to their mothers and Harry Harlow's wire mesh doll experiments with monkeys in the 1950s refuted both the Freudian and Pavlovian models of relationship.[25]

Science has only opened the doorway to understand human nature. Its best role is not to be a pontificating high priest, but to be a servant that provides insights and tools for human well-being.

Clarifying Human Nature and Readiness for Marriage

Correcting the confusion about human nature can help heal not only dysfunctional interpersonal relationships but also reform counterproductive societal and economic policies. Journalist David Brooks laments the failure to synthesize new research, which has allowed "[r]eliance on an overly simplistic view of human nature" to continue and lead public policy failures in education, health care, and foreign affairs. He highlights the fact that our society stresses development of hard skills while neglecting development of soft skills, which are moral and emotional in nature.[26]

Most Important Life Decisions

The family is where children learn about the nature of life, love and marriage, about human well-being, self-control, what is right and wrong, fair and unfair, who to make friends with and whom to oppose, and whom to marry and not marry.

What most Westerners are taught about love and marriage is that the happily-ever-after mental state of falling in love/romantic love is the benchmark and gold standard for marriage. It is deeply embedded in the American psyche.

Yet, the average person has difficulty talking about love, romance and marriage. Philosophers, social scientists and psychologists also have difficulty distinguishing "love" from sexual desire, liking a person, affection, and concern for others.[27] They also have difficulty taking seriously the association between romantic love and mental illness.

Anthropologist Helen Fisher with other neuroscientists used brain scanning machines, functional magnetic resonance imaging (fMRI), to study romantic love. They observed that the experience of falling in love suppresses areas of the brain that control critical thinking, produces a drug-induced "high" similar to addictive drugs such as cocaine, and a pathology associated with more negative emotions such as craving, anxiety, obsession, fear and thrill. [28] As neuroscientists describe, the mental state of romantic love is not voluntary, long-lasting or emotionally nurturing to the human mind and spirit or in relationships. It does not genuinely "mate" souls. It is like cocaine addiction and makes people "[love] sick" and "blinded by love."

In a forthcoming book we explain how the dominant belief of romantic love emerged from radical cultural changes in Western Europe and America. Also discussed is the mental health community's apparent lack of a framework to evaluate romantic love's negative side effects such as love sickness: loss of sleep and appetite, craving and withdrawal, heart fluttering, obsession and depression.

A healthy marriage is based on two mentally and emotionally healthy partners who premise their relationship on healthy beliefs about love and marriage.

(False) Romantic Love vs. True Romantic Love

Considering how deeply entrenched are the connotations of romantic love and falling in love in the Western psyche, in this book we call it (false) romantic love, to distinguish it from true romantic love--true love and romance within marriage, a state of mind that requires effort to develop and is nourishing and long-lasting. So please remember, we are not anti-love, we are pro-true love. We are not anti-romance, rather we are pro-true romance.

We have debated whether to use the adjective "true" before love because there is a widespread skeptical or cynical tendency engrained in our culture to presume that things in life are relative and to doubt anything that suggests being absolute. Widely accepted is the belief that all things of importance in human relationships last for only a short time—i.e., impermanence. The belief that true love waits, that one love is forever, and that true love is sacred, is fading.

Our definition of true includes that it is factually and morally correct, right, verifiable, realistic, consistent and ideal. True love in marriage, therefore, is lasting, sustainable, real and nurturing. It is not false, temporary, illusory, or destructive. So, there it is—true love.

Common Experiences:
Falling in Love, Mental Illness and Divorce

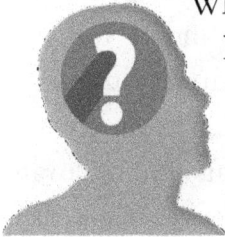

What does a mentally and emotionally healthy and an unhealthy person look like? Jason M. Satterfield, Director of Behavioral Medicine in the Division of General Internal Medicine at the University of California, San Francisco (UCSF), advises that while "there is no single prototype, there is a lot of overlap between them. In fact, it might be the same person at different points in his or her life." That is because "mental illness is common." "[O]ne in four people will have a diagnosable mental illness at some point in their lives."[29] And nearly 60% of adults with a mental illness did not receive mental health services in the previous year.[30]

Lack of care and treatment, the stigma our culture attaches to mental illness, and our misunderstanding of what mental health and mental illness are, contribute to America having among the highest rates of mental illness in the world.[31]

Brooks warns that America's health care policies will "…continue to fail unless the new knowledge about our true makeup is integrated more fully into the world of public policy…" [32] Seligman also brings attention to "misplaced government and industry priorities" in dealing with human health issues.[33]

There may be a public debate over health care policies and the nature of a healthy person, however, what do *you* think is a healthy human being and what does it have to do with being ready for marriage and forming a family? What do you think is healthy love? Those are serious questions.

When choosing a lifelong mate, you are predicting their future behavior as a husband or wife, and a father or mother (for those who desire to have children) "in sickness and in health." You are likely presuming that your mate will be your mate for a lifetime. But, how can you accurately predict and measure that?

Like mental illness, divorce is a common experience. While there may be debates whether the divorce rate is 41% to 50%, those odds of failure are very high.[34] And divorce can be a traumatic experience. So how good is your mate "picker?"

Predicting Behavior

Begin with some simple ideas that you may have heard before: a person's thoughts determine their behaviors, which determine their character, and their character determines their destiny. Cognitive behavioral therapy (CBT), a common psychotherapy, is similar in that it recognizes that thoughts (perceptions of events) influence a person's emotions and behaviors.

CBT therapists use Socratic questioning to help individuals learn to modify distorted beliefs to manage depression, anxiety, insomnia and other disorders.[35]

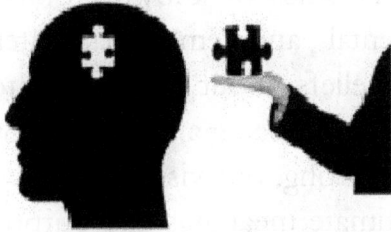

Many questions will be provided you throughout this book to think about the nature of a healthy human being who is able to form healthy relationships, and the realities of marriage and family life.

There are metaphors to comprehend how humans think and make decisions. One of them is a GPS (global positioning system), a navigation device, to describe a human's internal navigation system.

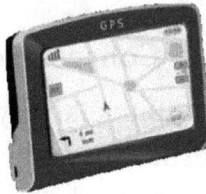

The Human GPS

Here is a quick review of that metaphor. Our van has a GPS with hardware and software to provide accurate digital maps for specific areas--depictions of streets, roadways and highways. If the maps are not accurate, they can lead us in the wrong direction or the GPS can default to a blank screen. After entering the address of our desired destination into a GPS, if we go off course or reach an obstacle that requires changing the route selected by the GPS, it will "intuitively recalculate" a different route to the desired destination. It keeps us on track.

Likewise, each human being has an internal GPS. At the "spiritual core" of our minds there is a kind of software

29

containing our faculties of knowing--spiritual intelligence, conscience, mental and emotional intelligence. Those faculties shape beliefs about love, ultimate meanings and purposes of life, about being a man or a woman, about self-worth, right and wrong, our vision for how to connect and realize those ultimate meanings and purposes, and how to live well. They shape how we navigate through life, make sense of it, form and maintain our relationships. They shape our character and provide the motivations for why we do things.

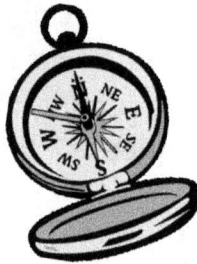

Conscience

Your internal GPS has an intuitive ability to recalculate your route to the desired destination when you go off course. It acts to keep you on track. Commonly it is thought to be your conscience that directs you to do what is right, like a *moral compass*. However, more is involved, because the conscience simply responds to what it understands to be right and wrong, true and false. There is a faculty of the mind that seeks out and informs your conscience of the greater good, with clarifications and corrections, as you make the effort to know the greater good.

Spiritual Intelligence

That faculty is spiritual intelligence, which is a religious/spiritual sensibility, a drive that seeks the higher good, the divine, God, things and sacred purposes, and universal principles. It makes us uniquely human. Spiritual intelligence guides, coordinates and integrates two other basic faculties of the mind--emotional and mental intelligence. It updates the conscience as well. Emotional intelligence seeks to know and do what is right in relation to others.

Spiritual Intelligence

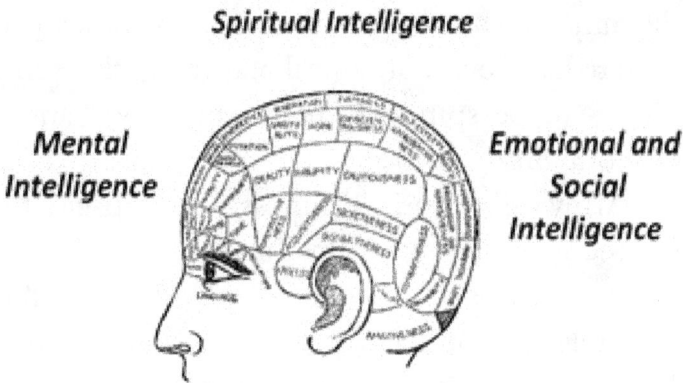

Mental Intelligence

Emotional and Social Intelligence

Educator Stephen R. Covey explains mental intelligence as the ability to see what is possible for oneself (vision), to sense one's calling (self-awareness), and to see what is possible for others.[36] While mental intelligence, and more recently emotional and social intelligence, are recognized as measures of human capability, spiritual intelligence is becoming more mainstream in research and discussion by scientists, philosophers and psychologists.[37] It can also poetically be called *heart*, considering its central importance.

Spiritual Fitness: Ability to Live by a Code Greater Than the Self

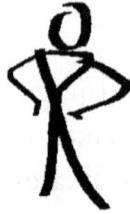

Spiritual intelligence is also becoming recognized as an important part of human well-being and performance. The Army recognizes that humans have a spiritual core, the foundation of the human spirit. Therefore, knowing that the dilemmas soldiers face in conflict zones are difficult and require high levels of ethical reasoning, the Army wants its soldiers to be spiritually fit, so they can "answer to a higher moral order."

The Army calls "spiritual fitness," the capacity to live by a code, the greater good, something that a soldier believes is greater than the self. The soldier determines their own personal religious or theological definition for the greater good. Spiritual fitness is necessary for soldiers and civilians alike and their families.[38] Indeed, the cohesiveness and health of a marriage, a family, any organization or society, depend upon its members living by a shared code of conduct that furthers its common good.

Coached by Seligman, the Army shifted its training focus from pathology to resilience and growth. The shift would help prevent PTSD, depression and addiction, and enable more soldiers to bounce back and be stronger.[39] In 2009, the Army initiated its *Comprehensive Soldier Fitness* program. It was designed to measure and strengthen the emotional, mental, social, moral and spiritual well-being of soldiers and their families.[40] In the beginning, the Army especially hoped that it would prevent PTSD and suicides that had begun to rise as soldiers served multiple tours in Iraq and Afghanistan. Later it transitioned into a general wellness program and was called the *Comprehensive Soldier and Family Fitness* program.[41]

Taking Seligman's advice, the Army recognized the positive correlation between higher levels of spirituality and lower levels of mental illness, lower substance abuse, more stable marriages, and greater resilience under high levels of stress in combat.[42]

Seligman's strategies help soldiers better prepare for the stresses of combat in conflict zones and convert post-traumatic stress into post-traumatic growth. Trauma can occur outside of conflict zones. It can also result from falling out of love or getting stuck in high-stress marital conflict. People do become love sick and heartbroken.

Several indicators in the Army's spiritual fitness module correlate with our Indicators for marital readiness that follow, such as self-mastery, resilience, humility, empathy and the capacity to live for purposes beyond self-interest.

Drive for Self-Transcendence

Similarly, Maslow concluded that there is an unselfish drive in humans toward self-transcendence. Also Erikson's and Vaillant's studies of human development confirmed that caring and living altruistically for the sake of others beyond one's self-interest promotes greater personal well-being.

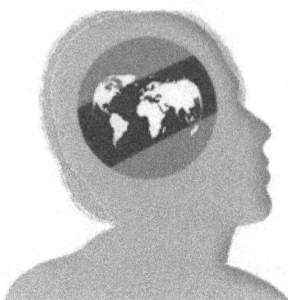

Spiritual intelligence informs the conscience of the greater good, when it is discovered through human effort. The maturity level of spiritual intelligence varies with each individual. As spiritual intelligence matures and connects with higher goods, universal principles, and the Divine, we humans are better able to know and trust in what is ultimately meaningful, to sense connectedness to the world and the universal purposes behind daily experiences and relationships. We are then better able to sustain commitments in the face of challenges and disappointments.

Therefore, the questions that follow are crafted to identify a potential mate's belief system (worldview)--what they understand to be the good, a good person, good relationships, and a good life. Marital readiness questions also seek to learn about a potential mate's personal beliefs about the purpose of marriage, whether it includes unselfish ideals beyond self-interest, and whether it is coherent or cherry-picked to justify particular behaviors.

Humility increases the capacity of spiritual intelligence by putting one's self and opinions into a larger context, the good and the greater good.

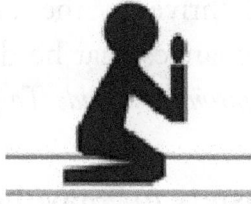

Real humility, though, does not mean being a doormat or hating oneself.

The Desire to Be Valued

Humans have the nature and desire to love and be loved, which also seeks transcendence. The reason that the counterfeit version of true love, that is (false) romantic love, is so powerful and euphoric is that it seeks transcendence. When the love impulse is directed toward wrong purposes, it is misused, dissipates, and leads to abuse, suffering and tragedy.

Humans also have the nature and desire to be good and seek the greater good, to be true and to seek trueness, to be beautiful and seek to be with people, things, ideas that are beautiful. Such desires are expressed through the powerful drive to collaborate and be recognized for the value that one contributes. The desire and capacity to collaborate is an important indicator of marriage readiness.

This human impulse is the driving force in the open-source community. At GitHub, the world's largest open-source community, programmers around the world contribute millions of hours of their labor for free and for only a little recognition for their creativity and efforts.

These human natures are probably at the root of journalist Thomas Friedman's optimism that humanity can adapt, survive and thrive in the face of supernova-like accelerating global changes that he describes in *Thank You for Being Late: An Optimist's Guide To Thriving In The Age Of Accelerations.*[43]

Self-Mastery to "Stay the Course"

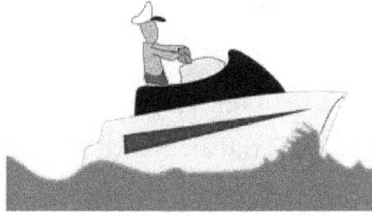

Marriage can enable human potential to be fulfilled. Wise psychologists, philosophers and religious thought leaders have advised that happiness is a by-product of unconditional and unselfish commitment to transcendent goods beyond self-interest.

A healthy adult possesses basic self-mastery, which is required for unconditional commitment. It is also known as self-management or self-regulation. Self-mastery is an ordinary ability, not an extraordinary ability, and can be defined as exercising basic self-control to subordinate bodily desires and unhealthy emotions to reason and moral values. It is a healthy habit of a "normal," socialized adult.

It is unfortunate that self-mastery is often considered an emotionally-loaded term. Even when self-mastery is regarded as the path to proficiency in the arts and sports, it is generally viewed as an extraordinary ability and possessed only by athletes and musicians who dedicate years to perfecting their skills. Even many religious people regard spiritual self-mastery as unrealistic and attainable for only a few. Images come to mind of an ascetic monk sitting on a block of ice in a Tibetan cave.

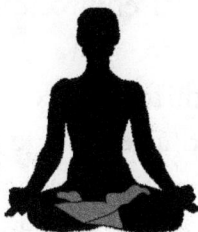

Jesus' call to "become as perfect as your heavenly Father is perfect" is regarded by many Christians as possible for Jesus but unrealistic for ordinary, sinful human beings.

The Executive Functions of Self-Mastery

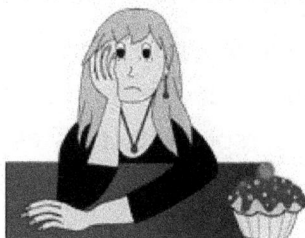

Self-mastery is not as extraordinary as it is commonly presumed; it is, in fact, necessary at each stage of human development to be healthy and to proceed to the next step of development. Self-mastery is the healthy exercise of "executive functions," which is a business metaphor used in neuropsychology to describe higher-level mental abilities and skills essential for learning, making healthy choices and achieving goals. These abilities enable us to remember, organize, plan, focus to control impulses, set goals and to achieve those goals.

We are born with the potential to develop them. We begin as children to learn these functions within our families and other social environments like schools, sports teams, and the workplace.

Self-mastery and different executive functions must be learned and developed at each age and stage of life to be a healthy functioning human being and to progress to the next stage of life. They are developed through disciplined routines, play, work, exercise, positive modeling and supportive family relationships.

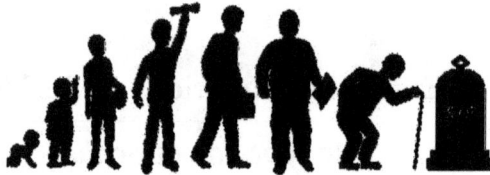

Self-mastery involves persistence and grit, self-discipline and impulse control necessary for commitment and for putting things in perspective. It is essential for empathetic listening and effective communication. Self-mastery means a high level of proficiency.

Self-Mastery in Marriage

When the daily requirements of marriage are considered, self-mastery is necessary to fulfill commitments, think and act compassionately, empathetically and skillfully to be a good team player. The ordinary challenges and intensity of married life can result in great stress, disappointments and frustrations due to misunderstandings, unrealistic expectations and unresolved dilemmas. Marriage is the most emotionally intense and intimate relationship in life.

Heaven or the greatest fulfillment and joy can be experienced in marriage. Self-mastery is necessary to develop true romance and the transcendence of becoming "as one" with one's spouse. Marriage offers the hope and opportunity to experience the most fulfilling of human emotions and desires.

Hell can also be experienced in marriage.

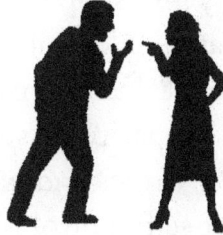

Intimate partner violence is a public health issue of epidemic proportions. Consider the fact that the American Academy of Family Physicians (AAFP) reports "[f]amily violence affects approximately a third of family physicians' patients."[44] "Nearly 3 in 10 women and 1 in 10 men in the United States have experienced rape, physical violence, and/or stalking by an intimate partner..."[45] Self-mastery is necessary to do no harm in marriage. Seeking to reaffirm that capacity, judges order abusive spouses to receive anger management classes.

When (false) romantic love is presumed to be the basis of marriage, self-mastery may not be considered a relevant idea. Following one's heart and feelings can mean just about anything, leaving young men and women ill prepared for marriage.

Ordinary Self-Mastery

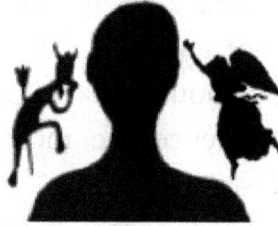

Basic self-mastery is simply management of one's impulses, emotions and actions in ordinary circumstances of life roles. Fulfillment and intimacy in marriage require personal mastery, the capacity to subordinate emotions of the moment to values, virtues and higher principles. That is not to say that perfect self-control is needed. Ordinary self-mastery is to have the emotional strength to be patient, to apologize, to forgive, to endure hardship, and to overcome disappointments and challenges for the greater good. Self-mastery is essential for healthy intimacy in marriage. It is an entry-level Indicator for marriage readiness.

What's the Big Deal?

You may be saying to yourself, "Why are they digressing about self-mastery, personal mastery or whatever you call it?" It is because drug addiction and other forms of substance abuse, pornography addiction, and domestic abuse are widespread problems in America's self-indulgent, overly-medicated culture.

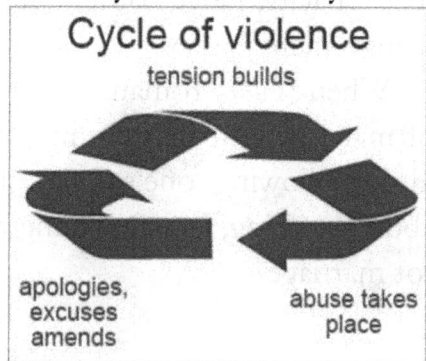

Cycle of violence
tension builds
apologies, excuses amends
abuse takes place

Able to Manage Emotions

Since responsible management of our emotions is important, let's take a closer look at emotions. They are conscious mental states that interpret and color life experiences. Emotions can help us to cope with and manage stress, or they can do the opposite. Emotions drive motivation that causes us to take action and to control our behavior. Emotions help us to identify how others feel and to respond with empathy.

Consider, for instance, the emotions of fear, anger and sadness. These emotions are felt when we interpret circumstances as threatening, violating our sense of justice, or when we are anticipating or suffering a loss.

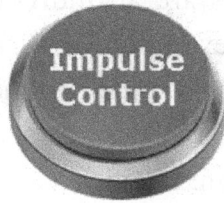

When those emotions are not managed and become out of proportion and distorted, they can lead to mental illness. When emotions like joy, personal pride and admiration of others are out of balance, they can lead to naïve detachment, arrogance and moral blindness. Emotions interpret life experiences through various filters, ways of knowing such as spiritual intelligence, emotional intelligence and mental intelligence.

Emotionally Fit for Marriage

How well one's emotions have matured and are managed influences whether one is emotionally fit and mature for marriage. Similar to the physical body, emotions

41

must develop and mature through stages to become healthy. Those who have experienced broken love affairs, a shattered engagement, or a marriage that ended in ashes, are challenged to recover and not withdraw into the shadows of depression and cynicism.

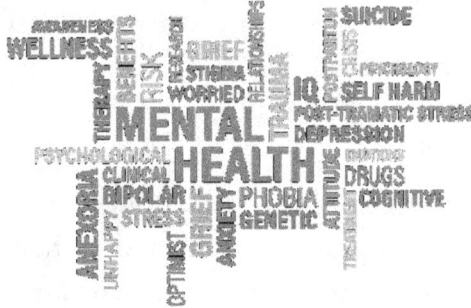

Scientists and academics distinguish between emotions and feelings. Feelings are an individual's internal *perceptions* of emotions. For example, the feeling (perception) of oneness, of being profoundly connected, emotionally and spiritually, is deeply satisfying. It satisfies the desires to be understood, appreciated and accepted for one's strengths and weaknesses, hopes, dreams, and fears. The feelings (perceptions) of emotional closeness and deep connectedness strengthen the bonds of commitments, enhance stability, nurture the human soul, and stimulate creativity and altruism. The feelings of alienation and being violated do the opposite.

Know Thyself

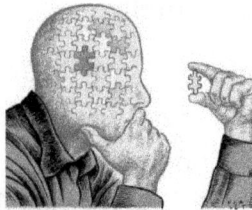

Self-mastery is more than mere self-dominance. It includes the capacity to be aware of one's self, emotions and feelings, and what one should do in the many roles of life.

Sense of Calling

Self-mastery also includes a sense of calling that develops through self-reflection and understanding the meanings of life. It is a drive to realize worthwhile life purposes and potentials that result in happiness and joy.

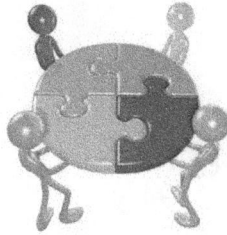

Sense of Connection

MIT professor Peter Senge said that attaining personal mastery (self-mastery) has no shortcuts or "quick fixes." It may take a lifetime to attain. Personal mastery encourages people to care for others. Also, individuals who exercise personal mastery see the connections in their surroundings and perceive everything as a whole.[46]

These unities of the self, the mind and body, and connections with others are expressed in Carl Jung's "Analytic Psychology," and Seligman's "Positive Psychology."

Creating a Framework for Assessment

Clarifying human nature and basic life principles will help identify the indicators of a basically healthy adult who is prepared for marriage. When they are shaped into checklists, they can serve as a basis for discussion and guide you through a process to make informed marital decisions. Such checklists are provided in the next chapters.

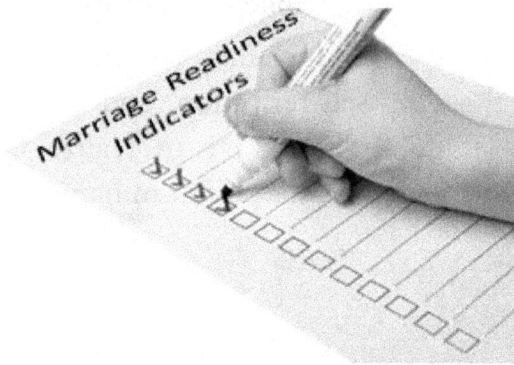

CHAPTER 3

Step 1: Preparation--
Identify Benchmarks And Indicators
Of Marital Readiness--
Benchmark One

"[True] love is an unconditional commitment to an imperfect person. To [genuinely] love somebody isn't just a strong feeling. It is a decision, a judgment, and a promise." – Unknown

Indicators
Autobiography
Biography
Benchmarking
Best Practices
Assessments
Plan
7 Steps

In this and the following two chapters, Three Benchmarks for marriage readiness and their predictive Indicators are explained. They are premised on evidence-based research about marriage, human well-being and family development, and provide a flexible framework of guidelines that you can tailor to your priorities and family traditions. These Three Benchmarks and Indicators provide concepts and a vocabulary to think and talk about the essentials of marriage. They touch upon different dimensions of ordinary self-mastery.

Three Benchmarks for Marital Readiness

A good marriage is based on how you treat one another *after* you marry. If your goal is a healthy, happy, nurturing marriage that lasts a lifetime, you need some basic capacities or proficiencies that can be called "benchmarks." When evaluating an individual's preparedness for marriage, whether of your "self" or of another individual, you are predicting how that person will treat their marriage partner after they marry. Predictions are based on their "entry-level" capacity and potential to meet these benchmarks. Three essential, entry-level capacities stand out. The capacity to:

1. Fulfill unconditional commitments,
2. Develop emotional and spiritual connection (intimacy), and
3. Creatively and interdependently collaborate.

Let us call them the "Three Benchmarks" and they are interrelated.

Indicators

Answers to relevant questions—Indicators--can help to predict how well a candidate for marriage matches up with each of the Three Benchmarks. They can reveal what an individual thinks, feels, and does. The questions that follow in the chapters consider the nature of a healthy human being and healthy relationships. They address a spectrum of factors such as an individual's sense of meaningful life purposes, love, courage, fairness, empathy, optimism, their ways of dealing with conflict and challenge, stress and forgiveness. Such questions are central to marriage and family and a cohesive, ethical society.

The Indicators are not calibrated to identify a "perfect" soulmate who would satisfy their spouse's every need, but rather to indicate whether an individual has the potential to fulfill the Three Benchmarks--basic, entry-level readiness to begin a life journey in marriage.

Patterns of beliefs and behaviors can emerge from an individual's Indicator answers, which suggest their character and personality and can predict their future behavior. As you step forward through the 7-Step Family Approach, verification of a marital candidate's answers can be done in layers.

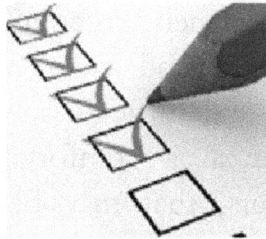

Some people may think that evaluating one's self and a potential marriage partner through the lens of the Three Benchmarks and Indicators that follow is "unromantic." However, they address very relevant issues and questions, whether one forms a marriage before or after one "falls out of love," by way of self-matching, by way of an arranged marriage, or through a family approach that we advocate. Marriage is a serious decision which requires thoughtfulness. If these Three Benchmarks and Indicators were considered as "essentials" in one's checklist of qualities for an ideal spouse, they could change the way people think about the nature of love, marriage and family. They are the fundamentals of commitment, intimacy and high-level teamwork to maintain and develop during marriage.

Begin with Realistic Expectations

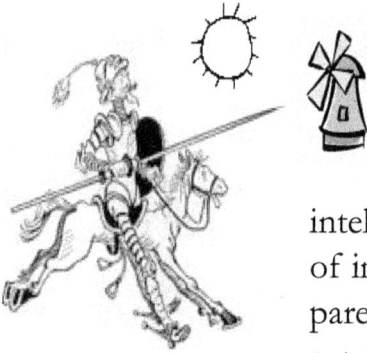

It is important to put marriage as a forethought and not as an afterthought. Indeed, the emotional, social, intellectual, and spiritual demands of interdependence in marriage and parenting usually far exceed the expectations that a young man and woman may have when entering into marriage. The demands of marriage and child rearing are great and present challenges and difficulties, which are not always pleasant nor occur at a comfortable pace. For naïve, perfectionist thinkers, that may be surprising. Ask any young couple with a few years of marriage under their belt.

Don't marry a fixer-upper (a real estate term describing a house for sale in need of major repairs). While marriage and parenting provide character-building experiences, they are not the places to attempt "to get one's act together" and become a responsible adult. That must be achieved before getting married.

Prevent Unrealistic Expectations

Another way of looking at this family approach to marriage is to ask whether it is reasonable that preparing for marriage and selecting a marriage partner deserve at least the same thought and effort as preparing for and selecting a college, a career, a car, a vacation location, a new phone, or a computer. Is marriage not even more important than these concerns and does it not therefore deserve more thought, effort and preparation?

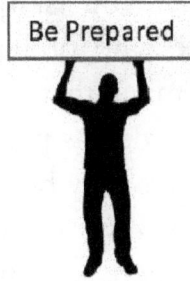

Be Prepared

A common mistake of young people is to fashion unrealistic expectations for both their career choices and marriage.

Prepare in Advance

There is always something new to learn when evaluating a person's readiness for marriage. Discovering the inner character of even close family members and friends that you have known for years occurs in layers. Therefore, it is important to reflect and prepare in advance your list of questions for your interviews.

Questions may be presented in a "Yes" or "No" format, or may be descriptive in nature:

- On a scale of 1 to 5, with 5 being the highest agreement, do you…;
- Please answer whether this statement is Very much like me ___; like me ___; neutral ___; unlike me ___: very much unlike me ___.

You may find it helpful to practice asking your questions prior to the interview and in a manner that helps facilitate the feeling of a natural conversation. Do your best to put a marriage candidate at ease so your questions do not feel like an interrogation.

The manner in which you ask questions is important. If you are the quiet type who prefers to think a lot before saying anything, remember that at some point your quiet reflection might be regarded as painful silence. Keep this in mind because a candidate may be that way, too. Therefore, observe how candidates reply to your questions, and don't jump to conclusions if there are long pauses in their replies.

What follows are Indicator questions for each Benchmark. They can help distill the meanings within the stories in the biographies that parents write about their son or daughter hoping to marry, and the autobiographies of those hoping to marry. The questions can serve as a guide during interviews and discussions with potential marriage partners and their parents. Don't be overwhelmed by the lists of questions. Use them selectively, as needed.

Benchmark One: Capacity to Fulfill Unconditional Commitments

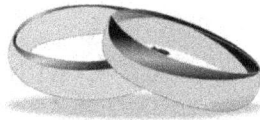

Commitment is important in marriage...and not just any kind of commitment--it is *unconditional* commitment. Yes, unconditional! No strings attached, without preconditions, and beyond a form of commitment that extends for limited periods of time, such as for every three to five years (serial monogamy). Unconditional commitment is for a lifetime in marriage. When the duration of marital commitment is dependent on the thrill of in-love feelings, one's marriage can evaporate like smoke.

In addition to a promise to remain married for a lifetime, unconditional commitment in marriage has many other dimensions: among them are to 1) do no harm to your spouse, 2) respect your spouse in public and private, 3) support the highest well-being of your spouse, for instance, health, education and vocation, 4) uphold the ideal and permanence of the social institution of your marriage, 5) seek the deeply intimate, transcendent unity of your marriage, 6) respect your parents and parents-in-law, 7) exemplify a healthy marriage and parenting before your children, 8) socialize your children to fulfill their adult roles in society, and 9) preserve, enhance, and perpetuate the "best of life" to next generations.

We have created a series of questions that seek to address such issues as the purpose of life and marriage, spirituality, stress management and conflict resolution, optimism, humility, manners, and more.

A Safety Net

Paul Amato, a family scholar, provides a useful definition for marital commitment: it is the "extent to which people hold long-term perspectives on their marriages, make sacrifices for their relationships, take steps to maintain and strengthen the cohesiveness of their unions, and stay with their spouses even when their marriages are not rewarding."[47] Making sacrifices for others means that there are values and virtues beyond the immediate individual happiness of each spouse, and obligations to others that are ended "only under the most extreme circumstances."

We agree with family scholars, such as Amato, who confirm that "commitment provides a mechanism not only to maintain marital stability, but also to recover from periods of unhappiness…. [and that] commitment also can strengthen happiness over the long haul."[48] It is a safety net.

Every couple is challenged to learn to love and adjust to one another and to *become* soulmates. Enduring feelings of affection and admiration can develop over time on the foundation of commitment. Mature and nurturing true love is a *decision* to fulfill virtuous purposes beyond how one feels in the moment.

Unconditional commitment is understandably an intimidating concept for many people, especially Peter Pan types. However, it becomes much more appealing with the understanding that personal happiness is in fact a by-product of such commitment. It is a precondition for a couple to trust one another, to take the risk of becoming emotionally, physically and spiritually united, to become "as one." Unconditional commitment is a precondition for a couple to free their minds to creatively cooperate to successfully transcend life's daily challenges. It is to do whatever is necessary for your marriage to survive and thrive. It is a measure of trustworthiness. Marriage is a shared, sacred commitment by a husband and wife who as equals support one another to realize personal excellence and fulfillment and to become "as one"—true soulmates.

Flexible and Not Blind

However, does unconditional commitment mean to unreservedly accept any abuse for any period of time? Of course not! At the same time, do married couples always measure up to their fondest ideals? No! And do they sometimes hurt one another? Yes! Unfortunately, there are many reasons for that. Whatever the reason, if you are the cause of harm, the ability to apologize, to make good faith efforts to correct your behavior, and to restore what was lost, like trust, are part of a healthy marriage and unconditionality. On the other hand, if you have been hurt, forgiving is a vital part of a healthy marriage, and prudent self-care. Genuine unconditionality is flexible and not blind. Marriages are regularly in need of repair, healing and restoration.

Indicators of Unconditional Commitment Motivations--What's in Your GPS Software?

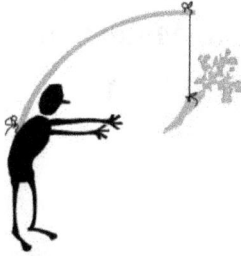

The strength of a person's commitments depends to a great extent on their motivations and ultimate loyalties. The factors that motivate commitment influence their resilience to stay the course in marriage and the quality of their marital experience. Search for the reasons that motivate you, your children, or potential mates to fulfill the various types of unconditional commitments in marriage. A boat captain must trust in a compass or GPS to navigate through both calm and stormy weather to the safety of a harbor.

Understand the content of a person's internal GPS software, and how well they, as the captain of their ship, could navigate through life.

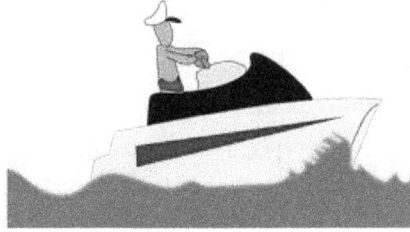

Consider asking:

- What is most important to you in your life, your priorities? What do you expect out of life?
- What is your vision for life? How does marriage and family fit into it?

Beliefs Can Make You Sick or Well

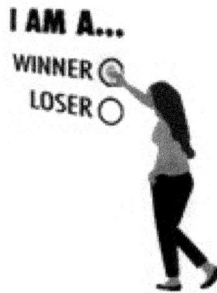

Most people recognize the existence of a mind-body connection. The Mayo Clinic cites surveys indicating "94% of patients regard their spiritual health and their physical health as equally important." A similar percentage of family physicians agree that spiritual health is important.[49] Beliefs are not merely words or thoughts. They affect how your body acts and can literally make you well or sick. Beliefs are connected with your entire being. The beliefs and purposes that your love impulses seek determine whether that type of love will nurture or make you sick.

Many Westerners marry because they feel that the overwhelming passion of falling and being in love is the unquestionable basis for marriage. They may feel that their marriage was founded in heaven and predestined by God. A reality check, though, would ask them whether their feelings of (false) romantic love and euphoric expectations can sustain a marriage for a lifetime. Is their marriage built on sand or rock? If the constant pursuit of uncomplicated delight and thrill is a couple's ultimate loyalty, they may feel justified to separate and divorce when their pleasurable feelings are no longer there. It is important to understand the foundation upon which a marriage is built.

People marry for other religious, spiritual, ethical, social, family reasons. Some couples are motivated by a belief that through marriage their personal fulfillment and human potential will be realized. That ideal may be expressed in religious language like developing a God-centered marriage, or spiritual language like achieving a transcendent oneness.

Altruistic beliefs are good for your health and your marriage. When couples share a spiritual belief in noble purposes greater than their self-interests, their inner lives can be enriched. Their individual uniqueness is not lost. It has been enhanced. Senge observes that people with self-mastery "have a special sense of purpose that lies behind their visions and goals.... They feel connected to others and to life itself."[50]

Desire to Live a Purposeful Life

Meaning questions that marital candidates might be asked are:

- What values/virtues do you deeply believe in? Why so?
- What is of utmost importance that instills the greatest meaning for you? Please describe personal experiences that demonstrate that.
- Do you believe in a higher power? If so, please explain. If not, please explain.
- In what do you ultimately trust? Why?
- Is there anything sacred or of ultimate meaning that is greater than yourself? Please explain.
- What experiences have cultivated or shaped that awareness?
- What is(are) the purpose(s) of your life?
- What purposes are you willing to commit your life to? Why so?

Positive Spirituality: Sense of Connection

Many of the marriage fitness concepts and questions dealing with spirituality and virtues parallel those used by integrative (holistic) physicians and the US Army's *Comprehensive Soldier and Family Fitness* program, who recognize the importance of positive spirituality and physical well-being. [51] Spirituality is a person's "sense of connection," that space between one's self and others-- your family, friends, other humans, nature, the universe, the higher power and ultimate meanings, virtues and principles. That connection instills a sense of personal identity and purpose for living. More questions that you could ask are:

- Do you find meaning in connecting with something larger than yourself?
- How do you describe your sense of what is sacred?
- How do you experience the sacred/the Divine: for instance, through nature, service to others, community, prayer, meditation, walking, worship, sports, music, other?
- What principles, beliefs, values or virtues beyond your family and other institutions or groups provide you with a sense of who you are and your life purpose?
- Describe how you perceive your spirituality and/or relationship with the ultimate Reality (the Divine, God, nature, other, etc.).

Calling

The ability to make recalculations when you get off track is related to positive spirituality and self-mastery. Senge has observed that those with self-mastery "...have a special sense of purpose that lies behind their visions and goals." [52] Having a conscious or intuitive vision of life purpose and direction provides a reference point to check your current path in life. Possible questions to ask are:

- Do you have a calling in life? If so, what is it?
- What do you really love doing? How does that relate to your ultimate meanings?
- What virtues do you deeply believe in? What contribution do you desire to make in life? What would make your work or school more meaningful for you? How does marriage relate to those desires?
- Are you true to your "self?"

Meaning and Purpose of Love and Marriage

How a person understands the purpose(s) of marriage and the nature of true love within marriage influences the scope of their marital commitments and how a husband and wife relate to one another. Questions relevant to the meaning and purpose of marriage are:

- Is there anything that you know that you should be doing but are not doing?
- Why do you want to marry?
- What is the purpose of marriage?
- What types of commitments are you willing to make in marriage?
- What is true love in marriage and how is it experienced?
- What are the stages of marriage?
- Is true marital love only a pleasurable feeling? When it is gone, what then?
- Is marriage only a private arrangement for personal pleasure?
- What do you want your marriage to look like?

Many unmarried men and women are stopped dead in their tracks by such questions. By default, their typical replies may be, "We want to be together. We know how we feel about one another. We love one another!" However, do they really believe commitment is "in sickness and in health" and "till death do us part"? Here is an interesting question:

- Do you believe that you will be together with your spouse even after physical death?

Today couples expect more from marriage in terms of emotional fulfillment. This is observed in both Western cultures and among urban, educated, upwardly mobile, middle class young couples in emerging economies like India. Many are less willing to tolerate differences and conflict, and less willing to make efforts to reconcile conflicts. Divorce is more acceptable to them and they view escape as the solution to marital problems.[53] They may presume that marriage should be an endless salad bar of pleasurable feelings. Also, they may be less committed to the institution of marriage, perceiving marriage as "just a piece of paper." At the same time, though, marriage is desired by most people and is increasingly regarded as a social status, a capstone or badge of honor, signifying that they have arrived at financial and emotional maturity. It is often publicly demonstrated through a big, expensive, blowout wedding.

From Me to We

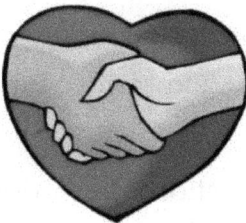

A healthy marriage is an intensely intimate experience. It involves a thoughtful, willful, disciplined and very emotional effort to move from "me" to "we." Through the partnership of marriage, a man and woman each can achieve a level of maturity, character development, intimacy, happiness and harmony that they could not achieve as individuals. Central to the sustainability of a marriage is whether the object of one's love is centered on "me" or on "we."

Marriage is more than an exclusively private arrangement for personal satisfaction. It includes purposes greater than the self: among them are the well-being of your spouse, your marriage, your children and your parents, and your extended family and society. They are compromised if you, your spouse and family become dysfunctional. More marriage related questions to consider are:

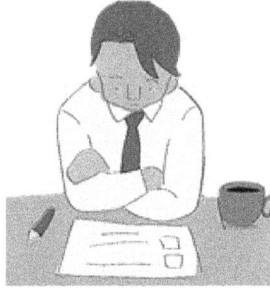

- How does marriage relate to your ultimate goods?
- What experiences shaped your concept of marriage?
- What are the vows/promises to which you will commit in marriage? What do these vows mean?
- How will marriage change you and your future spouse?

Some singles may think that the questions here don't apply to them, or that they are too difficult to answer. Whether before or after marrying, the questions are unavoidable. They are better asked before marriage rather than afterward.

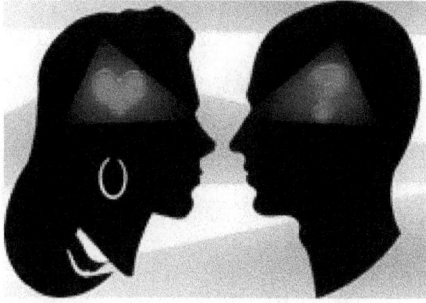

An important issue for single adults considering one another as a marriage partner is whether they can develop a shared vision for life, prioritizing their relationship above their careers. If they cannot, intimacy would be delayed or compromised. Career-focused men and women may postpone marriage, or if married, even regard their spouses as obstacles to their career success.

Resilience to Stay the Course: Love Fitness

Resilience is a big idea among health care providers who know that a strong immune system strengthens your resilience against disease and physical illness. Similarly, the *Army's Comprehensive Soldier and Family Fitness* program recognizes that a strong spiritual core is central to resilience and maintaining mental, emotional, and spiritual health. Resilience is the capacity to bounce back quickly from disease or difficulties. It is a spiritual immune system. It makes sense to incorporate resilience into the measurement of marital readiness and fitness.

Biographies, autobiographies and interviews can be used to verify and predict whether young men and women have love fitness, the resilience to "stay the course" of commitment, and to maintain high levels of caring, empathy, and partnership in marriage. Layers of questions add to 360-degree insights. Resilience-related questions to consider are:

- Do you make and keep your promises with your parents, siblings, and friends? Please provide examples.
- At school do you complete your assignments diligently and on time? Please provide examples.
- Do you take care of those for whom you are responsible? Please provide examples.
- At work are you a reliable employee: e.g., do you arrive at work on time, dress appropriately, get along well with fellow employees, have a good work ethic? Please provide examples.
- Are your words and deeds the same with your friends? Please explain.

Stress Management

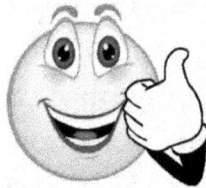

Related to building resilience is how well one is able to manage stress. In *The Worry Solution*, Dr. Martin Rossman, an integrative physician, explains, "Learning to manage stress is perhaps one of the most critical choices you can make in order to enjoy a healthy, productive life."[54]

There are many challenges that a couple faces in the course of marriage. High levels of *unrelieved stress* cause both physical and mental illness. It is recognized as a "significant risk factor" for a long list of illnesses such as heart disease, stroke, chronic pain syndrome, insomnia, and asthma.[55]

Stress is the unconscious, instinctual and instant physical response to a threat that originates from the most primitive, lower level part of our brain, the reptilian brain. When we stress about things that threaten us, and that we worry (think) about, signals are sent to that part of the brain, which activate fear and the fight-or-flight response.

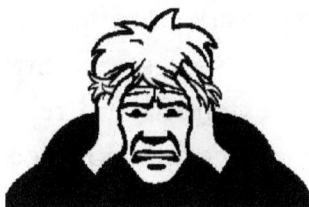

Stress can also be defined as something that happens to us. In our modern world, the main sources of stress are not physical dangers like a lion chasing us but are due to such things as loss of our jobs, money, relationships (quarrels, marriage, divorce, death of a loved one), and emotional problems (anger, resentment, guilt). When we perceive the demands of those stressors to exceed our resources, they cause anxiety, the *feeling* of apprehension or dread of a threat.

More than "20 percent of Americans (60 million) have diagnosable anxiety disorders," such as generalized anxiety disorder (GAD), panic disorder (PD), social anxiety disorder, phobias, obsessive-compulsive-disorder (OCD), post-traumatic stress disorder (PTSD), various depressions. Another 20 plus percent (60 to 100 million) of Americans have destructive habits or addictions like alcoholism, smoking, drug addiction, or eating disorders.[56]

On the other hand, well-managed stress and worry can also be a source of personal growth. We can use our higher-level brain centers and draw upon our underutilized emotional, spiritual and intuitive intelligence to manage worry, fear and anxiety. The Army's *Comprehensive Soldier and Family Fitness* programs, and integrative medicine are learning and teaching people how to do that.

For soldiers in war zones communicating with their families who are stateside, conflict at home can aggravate their already high levels of stress. Stress can take a heavy toll. The impact of extended and repeated deployments in Afghanistan, Iraq, and other conflict zones have steadily increased the divorce rate in the military.[57]

Similarly, in civilian life, the workplace and home can be zones of intense stress. There are many challenges that a couple face in the course of marriage. However, if family stresses are well managed, the bonds and health of a family can be strengthened.

During the Great Recession and the period immediately following, there was a heightened threat of losing one's job or losing one's home. If you know families who were on the verge of losing their homes and were being strung out by their lenders who were continually telling them that their loan modification request packages were not received or were lost, you know the protracted stress that can either pull a couple apart or be a uniting force. If family stresses are well-managed, the bonds and health of a family can be strengthened. Stress management questions to reflect upon are:

- What do you worry about?

- How do you manage stress at home, school or at work? Please provide examples.
- When something bad happens, how do you manage your emotions?

- What are your greatest sources of stress?
- How do you deal with them?
- What gets you upset?
- No matter how wise you may be, there are uncertainties in life beyond your control and are unresolvable. How do you deal with them?
- Disorders: Do you have any kind of physical, mental, emotional, or spiritual disorder?
- Do you have any "crazy buttons?"
- Do you drink alcohol? How often?
- How many drinks does it take before you become intoxicated?
- Why do you drink? Do you drive after drinking alcohol?

Ordinary Self-Mastery

Skillfully managing stress and developing resilience require the exercise of ordinary self-mastery, the mindful and conscientious control of one's emotions and behaviors. Having the emotional, mental and spiritual resilience to be patient, to apologize, to forgive, to endure hardship, and to overcome disappointments and challenges, is necessary in marriage. Positive psychologists have determined that self-mastery is a very good predictor of well-being and career success. Unlike inborn intelligence, it can be developed and improved.[58] Self-mastery is further defined in the previous chapter. Consider these questions:

- Does any of your family members drink excessively? Is any family member an alcoholic?
- Have you thought about how your drinking might affect your future marriage?
- Can you stand apart from your thoughts and feelings, and observe them?
- Can you change your thoughts and feelings?
- How well are you able to think ahead?
- Is there a habit that you would like to change but have not been able to?
- Are your moods regular? Do you have sudden mood swings? If so, do you know the reason (e.g., diet, stress)?
- How well do you control your temper when you get mad?
- During your childhood, did you get into fights?
- Have you ever had to apologize?
- Do you sometimes yell at people?
- How do you respond to disappointments? Please provide examples.

Reconciling Daily Dilemmas

Managing the complexities of life and daily dilemmas is challenging and unavoidable. It is advisable to examine how you and a prospective mate handle dilemmas.

There have been times when our van's GPS software did not work properly. It directed us south when we wanted to go north. That can occur when traveling through confusing big-city mazes of one-way streets and traffic jams.

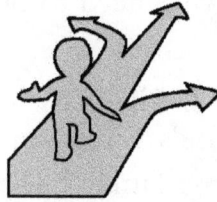

When that happened, we reset ourselves in the general direction that we knew was correct. Once we saw that the GPS had regained its senses, we continued relying on it for directions.

If we travel into areas beyond the scope of the GPS software, it is understandable why the navigation screen would become blank; for instance, if the software is programmed only for areas within the state and we travel into a different state. Updated software would then need to be downloaded. Or we could use an old-fashioned paper map. Or, yes, we could refer to a smartphone and see whether it does any better.

Similarly, there are times when the complexities and dilemmas of our lives are so confusing and intuition provides no quick and easy answers. We must pause, reflect, and sometimes brainstorm with others to sort things out. If we have a clear purpose and vision for our lives, we can maintain momentum and avoid the paralysis of analysis. Without a shared vision and purpose for marriage, dilemmas can pull a couple apart. *Me* can take precedence over *we,* and short-term gratification can subvert long-term well-being.

How one responds to those daily complexities and dilemmas is important. In today's economy and in large metropolitan and suburban areas near them, it is likely that both a husband and wife need to be employed to pay their basic family expenses.

There are many competing demands in a marriage: advancing each spouse's career, time to nurture intimacy, rearing kids, paying the family bills, and more. Reconciling them involves tough choices, especially when loss and disappointments occur. Questions relating to conflict resolution and resolving dilemmas include:

- How do you reconcile dilemmas with your parents, siblings, friends, and with colleagues at work? Please provide examples.

- Have you ever been frustrated or disillusioned by contradictions within your family, group of friends, your workplace, religious organization, country? When that happens, how do you respond; for example, say nothing, make sharp criticism, withdraw from the group?

- What will you do if you are not treated fairly among those groups?

- Every profession has a price to pay. Why do you think you could effectively manage the needs, stresses, and conflicts between your profession and your family?

- How will you know when your life is disordered with the wrong priorities...and is headed in the wrong direction causing you to neglect your health or your family?

- How will you reconcile the conflict of demands between your career, marriage and raising a family?

- How would you seek to put marriage at the level of importance that it deserves?

Humility

Humans make mistakes. Humility is required to admit our mistakes and to learn from them. There is not a lot of research on the subject of humility, although related subjects point to what it is not—narcissism, a disorder which has increased in recent decades.[59] Research on the subject of humility is impeded by the difficulties of defining and measuring it. A man may assert that he is humble, but in the eyes of others be seen as very arrogant and unaware of his offensive behavior. An honest and accurate view of one's self is needed.

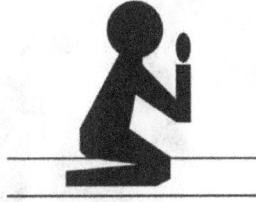

The benefits of humility are recognized as strengthened social bonds, improved health, and even better management of a high-performance organization.[60] For our purposes we define humility as a virtue, whether recognized in a religious, philosophical, moral or ethical context. Vanity, egotism and arrogance are its opposites.

Humility is a modest view of one's position and value in relation to others, ultimate meanings, principles, virtues, the divine, or God. True humility is honest and sincere. While recognizing the value of others, a humble person does not falsely deprecate their own value. Humility requires

69

constant openness, adherence to ultimate meanings, and self-awareness for self-improvement. Consider asking:

- What is the difference between arrogance and humility?
- How willing are you to admit that you are wrong about something? Please provide examples.
- How flexible are you in your approach to life? Please provide examples.
- Is it hard for you to forgive others and do you forgive yourself? Please provide examples.
- Do you tend to accuse people or are you reluctant to criticize others?

Whom Do You Trust?

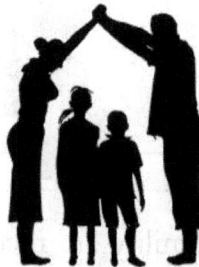

Humility, a modest and respectful view of one's position in relation to others, is related to trust. Trust in one's parents or those in parent-like positions is the bridge to receiving important knowledge, wisdom and traditions. Humility is recognition of the value and position of others. While the drive for ultimate meaning is innate, the capacity to govern one's life by a sense of the sacred and higher principles is shaped to a great extent by others, especially by one's parents in the early formative years. Parents impact our emotional, mental and spiritual health, even our physical health. Various medical studies report a correlation between parents who were warm and caring with their children's positive health indicators later in life. Those children had lower rates of risk for heart disease, cancer, and alcohol abuse.[61] If parents are caring and responsible, they can instill within their children the capacity to trust in relationships and in virtues and universal principles.

Therefore, it follows to be curious about whom a potential mate trusts and why. The answers to the following questions may be very helpful:

- Who do you trust to provide sound advice?
- What roles have your parents played in shaping your character?
- How has your internal guidance system (GPS) been influenced or shaped by your parents?
- What have you learned from your parents?
- What advice are you willing to receive from them?
- What advice are you not willing to receive from them?
- What values/virtues are most important to your family?
- In what ways do you want your future family to resemble the family in which you were raised?
- In what ways do you want your future family to be different?
- What family experiences or traditions shaped your sense of doing what is right in life?
- Do you express respect and admiration for your parents? How so? Please provide examples.

- Please describe the kindness expressed among your parents, grandparents, and siblings.
- Describe your evolution since childhood to live by values and virtues important to you.
- What role do you think your parents should play in the selection of your spouse and in your eventual marriage?
- Besides your parents, what other adults have you received important advice from (coaches, mentors, teachers, religious leaders, etc.)? What was it and why was it helpful?
- Do you have anyone that you can share your heart with, your hopes and fears?

Flexible Optimism

Unconditional commitment requires mental toughness and optimism, important measures of health. Optimism is the expectation that setbacks are temporary and that you will eventually succeed in life. Seligman found that optimists have strong resilience and bounce back quickly. Pessimists tend to think that their setbacks will last, that they will affect everything in their lives, and there is nothing that they can do about it. They tend to underachieve, become depressed, fail to bounce back, and have less stable relationships.[62]

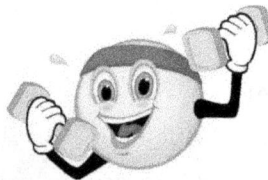

Seligman further defines optimism in its healthy form as "flexible optimism" that is guided by reasoned faith, and *not*

a blind habit…, which leads to destructive consequences. Do you know someone *with nothing more* than blind optimism who, after years of dead ends, asserts, "I am following my passion wherever it may lead me"? College commencement speakers often provide such advice to graduates. Your worldview provides filters through which life experiences are interpreted. Consider these optimism/pessimism questions:

- Are you optimistic about life? Your future? Why so?
- Is there an overriding goodness that prevails in life? If so, what is it?
- Considering the continual pattern of wars and inhumanity to man, do you believe that good will overcome evil. Why?

With a little thought, you can fashion questions that are best suited to the candidates that you are considering.

Modesty

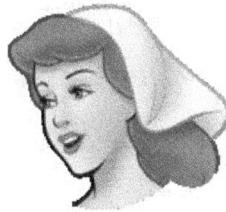

A modest person does not try to draw attention to themself in their speech, behavior or manner of dress. Yes, the standards of modesty vary by culture; however, what does modesty mean to you or a potential mate? Consider:

- What are examples of a modest person?

- How would you like your spouse to dress?
- Would you mind if your spouse used profanity? Why?
- How do you express modesty in your life?

Manners

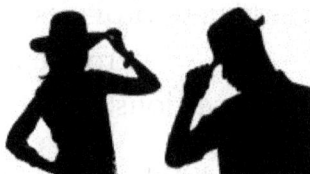

The habit of good manners expresses respect for others. It is the exercise of self-restraint and concern for others in everyday situations that comply with a code of expected behavior within a particular social group. Manners apply to hygiene, courtesy, and other social customs. How about these questions?

- What manners are important to you?
- What is a gentleman? What is he expected to do?
- What is a lady? What is she expected to do?
- What manners did your parents stress in your home?
- Is there something that your mother sometimes reminds you to do?
- When you meet a stranger who is older than you, how do you address them?

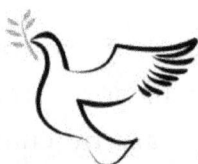

Chastity

Chastity has been discussed in earlier chapters. Consider asking a marital candidate:

- What is chastity? Is it a good thing or a bad thing?
- What is abstinence? Is it a good thing or a bad thing?
- What do you think about sex before marriage? Why so?
- Is sex before marriage okay? Why?
- Is it difficult to be abstinent before marriage?
- What do you think about flirting? Why?

Adversity & Disappointments

Related to resilience is how a person responds to adversity and disappointments. Possible questions are:

- How do you digest hardship?
- How do you approach unpleasant work?
- How do you respond when you are not understood or supported?
- How do you respond to disappointments?

Moral Courage (Chivalry)

We all have a hero

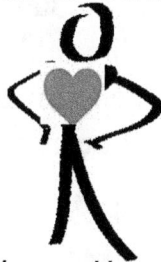

In our Heart

Courage–moral and physical--is a practical necessity while navigating through the economic, social and political uncertainties of our present-day world. Courage is acting according to virtues, to do what is right, and to help others in spite of potential opposition or personal risk of loss, whether it is physical, financial, or social. Courage is a mindset that is part of human nature. It does not mean taking action without fear, but rather despite it. Healthy amounts of fear are needed for survival.

In our country's public arenas, such as in politics, moral ambiguity prevails where people seem to no longer agree on what it means to be good or principled, or courageous. Courage is rarely linked with the private lives of individuals in their marriages and families.

Millions lost their jobs and homes during the Great Recession. Courage was required for fathers and mothers to stabilize their families and make new beginnings.

Consider pregnancy. Even with modern medicine, there are still risks of severe complications. It takes courage for a woman to give birth to a child. Pregnancy and birth are enormous life changes, which can be overwhelming. The stakes are high. When children become mature enough to be grateful, mothers are often fondly remembered as saintly heroes. The expectation of courage has been marginalized to fantasy heroes and elite athletes, and to those in the military, police, and fire departments.

Questions related to courage could include:

- How do you respond while experiencing sickness or adversity?
- Do you desire to have children? Why so?
- What changes do you think having children would cause for your life?

- What would you do if some calamity happened where all your finances were lost, or you lost your capacity to pursue your present career choice, or you lost your health, what would you do?
- If you lost your job and home, how would that impact your marriage and the well-being of your children?
- What are some examples of how one could act courageously to keep one's marriage and family together and live with dignity? How would that be possible?
- What are examples of you standing up for what you believe?
- Why did you act in this way?
- Where did you learn such behavior?

Chapter 4

Step 1: Preparation
Benchmark Two:
Capacity for Intimacy--Emotional
and Spiritual Connection

"When you show deep empathy toward others, their defensive energy goes down, and positive energy replaces it. That's when you can get more creative in solving problems."--Stephen R. Covey

A couple may intend to make unconditional commitments in marriage, however, if they do not have the entry-level capacity to develop lasting intimacy in marriage, they can become lonely, emotional strangers. Intimacy and love in marriage are profoundly misunderstood. Intimacy is commonly associated with mere physical closeness and the biological drive for sexual relations. *Lasting* intimacy and *true* love, though, are fundamentally about emotional and spiritual connection of the mind and heart.

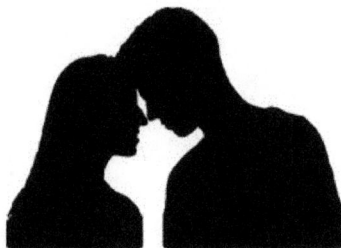

More Than Physical

Becoming "as one" in marriage is more than 3 to 13 minutes of sex--the range of "adequate" to "desirable" time for an orgasm and ejaculation to culminate during vaginal intercourse, which American and Canadian sex therapists believe is normal and not cause for clinical concern by couples.[63] That, of course, is the duration to climax for men. Women are different in physiology and nature from men; therefore, for those reasons and more, simultaneous climaxes between husbands and wives are not common, and more is involved for mutually satisfying intimate connection between a husband and wife.

Physical contact may seem like genuine intimacy for a while; however, lasting intimacy and true love do not magically occur merely when two bodies join together for sexual intercourse. Singles may think that such magic will happen because that is what happens in the movies, novels, and in popular music. Having sex is not the source, though, of lasting marital intimacy.

Reality talk show host Rabbi Shmuley Boteach argues that the Western concept of sexuality inhibits lasting passion and intimacy. He explains that it is excessively goal-oriented "—so strongly focused around sexual climax—that most of us scarcely know the benefits of a *means-oriented* sexuality. And it's killing both our marriages and our general enthusiasm for life. *Life is not meant to climax.* Climax is death." Also, when a husband's sexual climax is prioritized, it often leaves his wife's fulfillment neglected, which leads to overall marital dissatisfaction. Boteach affirms that when contrasting the sexual nature of men and women, men are quickly bored. "After sexual climax they're all but dead…. The history of relationships has been that the female need for attention has rarely been matched by the male attention span…"[64]

The Natures of Men and Women Are Different

Therefore, Boteach encourages men to understand the different anatomy, sexual nature and experience of women. He explains that changing "our lives from a goal- to a means-orientation would bring back the curiosity and passion that is the very stuff of the erotic spark." Also enjoying the journey of life and marriage and longing for your spouse would renew physical, emotional and spiritual intimacy. He advocates rejuvenating marriage with such practices as revitalizing innocence, novelty, curiosity, intelligent conversations, and women wearing modest clothing to enhance natural attraction.[65]

Sex Can Occur Without Genuine Intimacy

Sexual relations can occur without emotional or spiritual intimacy. Sadly, and all too often, after a blissful honeymoon period, couples continue to hold confusing and unrealistic expectations for love and intimacy. As a consequence, they may become emotional and spiritual strangers stuck in the land of "me," unable or unwilling to cross into the land of "we," where they can experience the greatest fulfillment.

Couples who are stuck in an emotional wasteland can end up drifting apart, experiencing loneliness, and hurt each other with criticism, contempt, defensiveness and stonewalling. The end result can be not only divorce, but often mental and emotional illness and physical violence. The tragic divorce and domestic violence rates indicate that often couples are not able to sustain healthy intimacy in their marriages.

If the character and interpersonal skill sets to develop emotional and spiritual connection do not exist before marriage and before having sexual relations, it will be more difficult to develop them afterward.

Lasting Intimacy

It is important to understand the nature of lasting intimacy in marriage. There is a universal desire among human beings to connect with people because our human nature is to love and be loved, the impulse to seek a relationship with an object of desire.

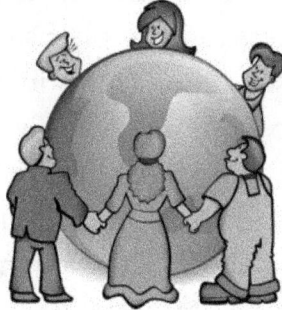

We crave intimacy and people are sensitive to being rejected and emotionally hurt.

In marriage, we seek a higher quality of emotional and spiritual connection. We are motivated by our drives for self-transcendence and transcendent union because we are spiritual beings, not just physical beings. The desire to be intimately "as one" with a beloved life partner is central to human nature and the human experience. Indeed, it predates the legal and religious definitions of a husband's and wife's "oneness," which originate in common law and Christian doctrine--"they shall become one flesh"— Genesis 2:24.

True and lasting intimacy in marriage is a by-product of true love. It is developed over time--it does not just effortlessly happen. True and lasting intimacy is sustained by the unselfish capacity to seek the utmost good of the other, to continually give and receive respect and safety, acceptance, friendship, forgiveness, attention, curiosity, appreciation, fondness and admiration. Indeed, more than periodic 3- to 13-minute episodes of sex are required to maintain a healthy marriage and lasting love.

Intimacy, Love, Sex Misunderstood

Deeply entrenched in the Western culture, psyche and mythology, intimacy, love and sex are misunderstood and falsely idealized. Increasing emphasis on individualism, self-actualization and self-gratification in the *pursuit of happiness* has contributed to a more radically individualistic rather than a family-centered society. Filial piety and reverence for marriage are not highly prioritized virtues. These cultural trends have earned the US the infamous reputation as a world leader in divorce.[66] Central to shaping today's divorce patterns is acceptance of (false) romantic love as the bedrock basis of a happy marriage, even though it is capricious and unstable in nature.

Sex and Intimacy Commercialized

Western entertainment industries have portrayed love as essentially physical and have linked intimacy with sexual relations by commercializing sex; the human body is objectified as a mere instrument of sexual pleasure, a commodity devoid of personality and dignity. With the 24/7 accessibility of pornography, men and women substitute fantasy pornographic images for their spouses and men replace intimacy with their wives with masturbation.

Even recent Disney animations, not older ones, have increasingly sexualized their characters, especially the princesses. Their figures (tiny waists, big busts), body movements and clothes of female characters like Jasmine (in *Aladdin*) and Ariel (*The Little Mermaid*) are sensual and sexually attractive. Children's imaginations are filled with these images and romantic, unrealistic expectations about love, sex, and male/female relationships. They are conditioned to think that true love and romance are represented by the Prince Charmings and their teenage princesses who fall in love at first sight; that you will know who is "the One"—your soulmate--because you will feel "it" as "chemistry"--excitement like electricity running through your body, butterflies in your stomach, craving and sleeplessness, magic and romance will surround you, and that you will live happily-ever-after with your soulmate.

The importance of intense feelings of excitement and passion in the mental state of (false) romantic love are overemphasized as the decisive factors in human relationships. They are exalted as the ideals and the basis for marriage. Consequently, when sexual passion and excitement fade in a marriage, couples presume that love has faded away into the distance and their marriage is unsustainable.

There is confusion and ambiguity about true love and intimacy, in part because the singular word "love" does not distinguish the feelings experienced between spouses, family members, friends, employees, citizens, or love for animate and inanimate things, ideas and music.

Counterfeit Transcendence

Western culture has narrowed and obscured the transcendent dimension of true love and intimacy in marriage by basing it in mythology, false ideals and unrealistic expectations.

Consider the soulmate myth. It has various origins. In Plato's *Symposium*, Zeus cuts in half androgynous humans who are half man and half woman. As two incomplete halves (souls) they "search" to "find" one another (their soulmate) to become whole persons, and when connected, they will immediately enjoy the ultimate human experience of climactic, euphoric love and live happily-ever-after. Their search is aided by an external supernatural force like Cupid or Love.

The soulmate myth also comes from religious/spiritual predestination views that marriages are made in heaven by a divine source.

Movies, music and novels perpetuate the soulmate myths because they are profitable and appeal to deep longings for emotional, transcendent, exclusive, and everlasting relationships. A fundamental reason that the falling in love/being in-love experience is essentially unquestioned is that it has a transcendent, intoxicating feeling to it.

The process and nature of becoming "as one" is falsely idealized. True intimacy does not just effortlessly happen; it is developed over time with personal investment and sacrifice. Marriage itself is a spiritual discipline to achieve self-transcendence and transcendent union. In marriage, true intimacy is the capacity to continually give and receive acceptance, empathy, forgiveness, one's attention, safety, appreciation, fondness and admiration.

Humans tend to overestimate what God, Cupid or the angels should do and underestimate what they should do.

Singles tend to romanticize love and intimacy into something that it is not. Their unrealistic expectations set them up for disappointment and suffering.

The Consequences
Increased Loneliness

While it may be argued that the Internet has enabled people to have a wider and more diverse communication with others, loneliness is a sad reality of modern life.[67] From Harvard sociologist Robert Putnam's *Bowling Alone*, to social neuroscience revealing that social contact is a biological drive, to Prime Minister Theresa May appointing a minister for loneliness,[68] feelings of social isolation are a global problem for millions of people in industrialized societies. In Western societies, people are spending more time online than in face-to-face communication.

Sadly, Americans, especially Millennials, are becoming lonelier,[69] the subjective feeling that they lack intimate connection with others: 12 to 23 percent of Americans "say they have nobody to talk to (in 1985 that figure was 8 percent)."[70] Consider asking:

- Do you find it difficult to talk with anyone that you can trust to listen to your hopes and concerns?

The "General Social Survey" reports that those who say that they have no friends have about tripled in number in recent decades.[71] And 60 percent of lonely people are identified as married.[72] This is consistent with divorce rates nearing 50 percent for first marriages and more than 60 percent for second marriages. You would think that after a divorce, the chances of another divorce would be lower.

However, "'remarried adults have a higher likelihood of divorce than those in their first marriage.'"[73] Additionally, growing older does not necessarily mean becoming wiser. By 2009, more Americans over age 50 were divorcing, and 53 percent of them divorcing at least a second time.[74]

Decline of Intimacy and
Sexual Frequency in Marriage

Not only are Americans becoming lonelier in our hyper-connected Internet age of Facebook and Twitter, and where sex and pornography are easily accessible, they are losing their passion for the most powerful physical intimacy–sexual intercourse.

A University of Chicago study reports that as American adults grow older, they are steadily losing their sexual desire. The study reveals that adults 18-29 have sexual intercourse 84 times per year, which declines to 63.5 time per year in their 40s, and further drops to 10 times per year for those 70+: "Among the married the decline is even more striking, dropping from 109 times per annum [note, though, frequency is still more than those unmarried] for those under 30 to 17 times per annum for those 70 and older…. even among couples who rate their marriages as very happy (GSS, 2005) and among those who say they are still 'in love' (Greeley, 1991) frequency of intercourse declines with age." Understandably, happily married couples have greater sexual frequency than those unhappily married.[75]

Several studies of erectile dysfunction (ED)--alternatively known as impotence--also report that its prevalence increases with age and is a common problem among men.

By age 40, 40% of men are affected by ED and it increases to about 70% for men in their 70s.

It is important to remember that while physical health problems such as diabetes contribute to ED, other psychosocial and emotional problems are significant causes of ED.[76]

Return to Medieval View of Love

Considering the sex-saturated culture that we live in, with loneliness increasing and complaints that marriage is boring, it is common today for Millennials and Gen Xers to cynically presume that sexual passion, excitement, discovery and creativity end after committing to marriage. Many presume that marriage becomes boring after a few years, and that one quickly knows everything there is to know about one's spouse and marriage. They are leaning to the presumption that true love exists outside of marriage.

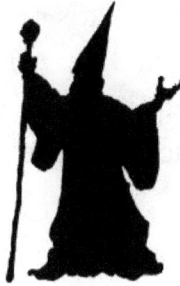

This pessimistic notion resembles the medieval literary view of courtly love that taught true love could only be experienced outside of marriage. Medieval romantic stories extolled the virtues of a superhero, a "lovesick" knight—a gentleman in shining armor (like Sir Lancelot)—who has an adulterous relationship with his boss's wife (King Arthur and Queen Guinevere). Western literature has been dominated by medieval romances, the stories of adventure, passion and adultery. They shape our popular culture's notions of love, marriage and romance, and tragically, sabotage the possibilities for true love and happiness.

Denis de Rougemont, a Swiss philosopher, famously concluded, "To judge by literature, adultery would seem to be one of the most remarkable of occupations in both Europe and America. Few are the novels that fail to allude to it…. Without adultery, what would happen to imaginative writing? Novels and plays subsist on the so-called 'breakdown of marriage'." He asks whether Westerners are attracted to what destroys marriage as much as to what strengthens it.[77] Is there a vicarious pleasure and charm about the forbidden?

The romantic myth that lovesickness and obsession are signs of true love is false. They are not good for your health. It would be just as faulty to presume that commitment to marriage leads to a loss of creativity and excitement, as it would be wrong to conclude that commitment to a startup business in hope of a prosperous future would automatically cause a loss of creativity and excitement.

Internet Porn Addiction

Increasing numbers of young and older males *and* females are turning to online pornography as a source of sexual excitement and novelty. Porn is available to them 24/7.

In 2014, the Barna Group determined that 79% of males 18 to 30 years old viewed pornography once per month and 63% viewed it more than once per week. Females in that age group had lower percentages, but they were still significant: 34% viewed pornography once per month and 19% viewed it more than once per week.[78]

The accessibility and diversity of pornography seduces many into fantasy relationships with unrealistic and degrading sexual images. Neuroscientific studies have found evidence that their brains are gradually rewired to be stimulated in specific ways by online porn. Dopamine is secreted in the brain with each click of the computer mouse and each visually stimulating and sexually gratifying encounter with pornographic images. Dopamine, which communicates to the body that it has done something pleasurable (perceived as a good), serves as a reinforcement for behavior--it encourages the brain to recall and repeat certain behaviors to reproduce pleasurable feelings. The act of seeking, such as surfing for porn, or seeking illicit sexual relationships and adultery, triggers the reward system. This helps explain why something that feels so good can be so bad. So, what is the harm of viewing pornography?

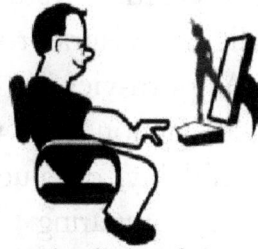

Lure of Excitement
Erectile Dysfunction

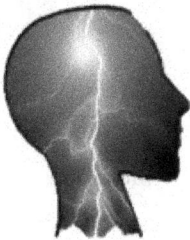

Studies reveal that young adult males exposed to pornography demonstrate more heartlessness, aggressiveness and violent attitudes toward women, such as regarding rape as less serious. With porn addiction, a husband's brain becomes less responsive to touching his real wife. She does not compare to the conditioned excitement of fantasy porn images of other women; he is not excited by her. Nor is his wife appreciated and satisfied. He is not aroused and can incur erectile dysfunction (ED).[79] That's good news for Cialis and Viagra profits, but bad news for the couple.

As porn-viewing males are more likely to express sexual dissatisfaction with their partner, they are more accepting of infidelity, devalue marriage and more likely to divorce. Males comparing their sexual experience with fantasy women can lose interest in actual women, which prevents them from forming healthy relationships with women.

Porn addiction can eventually create an overload of dopamine, which overrides normal satiation mechanisms and causes desensitization to dopamine. That can lead to depression, social anxiety, OCD and other mental health disorders.[80] Consider asking:

- Do you think viewing pornography is acceptable? Please explain.
- Do you view pornography? If so, how often?

Inconvenient Questions Left Unanswered

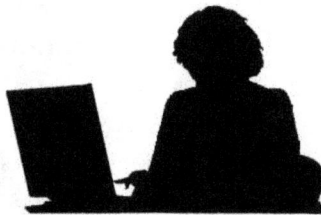

Large percentages of young males and females do think that viewing pornography is acceptable. Considering that, "inconvenient questions" left unasked and unanswered can later haunt and undermine a married couple's relationship.

Do you think that women are immune to the same damage? Women may think that they are immune, and that pornography would make loneliness seem normal and mask their insecurities. In her blog, Lauren Dubinsky explains why they are wrong. She shares her personal experiences and "wish list"--warnings of the damage to her from watching pornography that she wished she would have received before she started watching porn.[81]

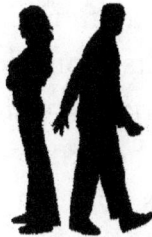

Comparing one's spouse with another person, whether the result of online porn addiction, or a romantic attraction, leads to dissatisfaction and a loss of intimacy. It emotionally pushes couples apart to seek appreciation, passion and excitement elsewhere.

Healthy Inner Lives
Healthy Practices

The studies that reveal increasing loneliness, boredom and declining sexual intercourse with age do not mean that sex automatically becomes boring with age. The reality is that the secret to sexual satisfaction resides between the left ear and the right ear (one's mind and brain—the most important sexual organ). The reality is that sex is as good as you make it; older can be very sexy. Surveys, for example, reveal that "the percentage of people 45 and older who consider their partners physically attractive increases with age."[82] Medications, vaginal lubricants and hormone creams can overcome many physical problems that impair sexual relations. Loneliness, long-term familiarity (boredom) and hurt in a marriage relationship can be offset by healthy emotional and spiritual practices.[83]

The intimacy of oneness in marriage can be deeply satisfying, but it must be learned, earned and developed if it is to last a lifetime. The issues for single adults considering one another for marriage relate to whether they have the entry-level capacities and skill sets to learn, earn and develop lasting intimacy in marriage.

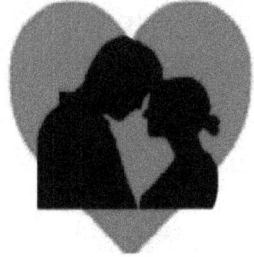

Earlier we discussed "spiritual fitness" and the need to live by a higher moral order, necessary ingredients for human well-being and for meeting the need for self-transcendence. In marriage, living virtuously and transcending one's self are essential—acting unselfishly, with care, honesty, empathy, gratitude and more.

Intimacy Indicators

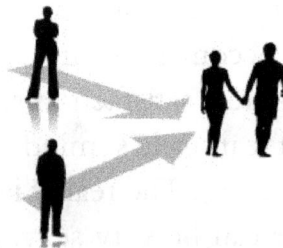

Maintaining a healthy emotional and spiritual connection in marriage requires each partner to manage a healthy inner life and to exercise basic self-mastery. A person's system of knowing--emotional, spiritual and mental intelligence, which directs how one navigates through life--must function properly. It is like your vehicle's GPS hardware and software, which, if functioning properly, knows

- where you are located (identity, self-awareness),
- correctly adjusts its directions (empathy, self-awareness, self-worth)
- so you can arrive at desired destinations (your life purposes, vision and calling).

A marital candidate's answers to Indicator questions can triangulate to suggest the health of their inner life and whether they have the capacity to emotionally and spiritually connect in their marriage.

Identity

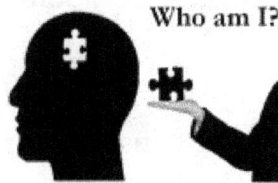

Who am I?

If an individual is confused about their identity (who am I?), has limited self-awareness, or does not have a healthy sense of self-respect and self-worth, they will have a difficult time navigating through life, especially with their spouse, whose well-being is interdependent with theirs. Consider these questions:

- If you were to introduced yourself to our family, how would you describe who you are?
- What has shaped your identity?
- How do you think your career will shape your identity or has shaped your identity?
- How do you experience your sacred center?
- Are you a different person today than you were 3 to 5 years ago? How so?
- Do you see yourself becoming a different person in the future? Please explain.
- Describe who you are and how that affects your relationship with others.
- What would it be like if you married someone just like yourself in terms of personality, temperament, and character? Would you like that?
- What gives you strength?

Self-Awareness
Self-Respect/Self-Worth

Personal self-awareness is related to one's ability to respect others, and to maintain healthy self-respect and self-worth irrespective of constant approval from others. A spouse with a diminished sense of self-worth may abuse their partner to falsely feel superior. Possible questions to ask are:

- When are you the happiest?
- When are you the most unhappy?
- In what form do you like to receive love (e.g., touch, gifts, words of encouragement, time together, etc.)?

- Is your manner of making decisions predictable? How would you describe it?
- What do you do or say that indicates you are self-aware?
- Do you like yourself? Why or why not?
- Deep down, do you feel that you are a person of value? That you count?
- Do you feel wanted and accepted? By whom?
- How competent do you feel about yourself in what you do in work/school?
- Describe the basis of your sense of self-worth. Does it depend on how others respond to you?
- Does your sense of self-worth depend upon your grades in school, what you produce (salary, other) at work?
- Do you need immediate positive feedback to have your self-esteem affirmed?
- Are you true to yourself?

Vision: Where are you going?

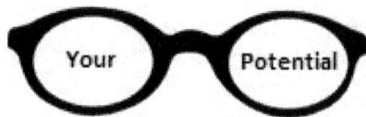

Covey regards the highest manifestation of mental intelligence as vision and a healthy sense of self—seeing what is possible in yourself and in others.[84] If a person has little sense of positive purpose, value and possibility for him/herself, or for anyone beyond themselves, their personal well-being and that of others is likely to be neglected or misdirected. Recognizing that the path to personal fulfillment is interconnected with the well-being of others is vital. The following questions could be asked. Some are mirrored in Benchmark One, however consider them in the context of Benchmark Two:

- Where do you see yourself in 5, 10, 20 years? Do you have a vision or calling for your life?
- What is your passion and your ambitions?
- Do you hope that your spouse will share your ambition?
- What have you always loved doing?
- What do you care deeply about that is happening in your family or at work or school?
- How do you see marriage fitting into your life?
- What does marriage have to do with your personal development?
- When are you at your best?
- What unique talents or abilities are you really good at?
- When are you at your worst?
- What accomplishments in your life are you most proud of?
- What opportunities do you see for your growth and development?
- What efforts are you making toward self-development?
- How do you attempt to learn from mistakes?
- How important is artistic expression for you? Is it central or peripheral to your life?
- What are your greatest unmet needs right now?

- If you could do one thing that would create the highest value in your life now, what would it be?
- What habit or habits would you like to change?
- What is your greatest source of stress?

Stepping Stones for Emotional Connection, Empathy and Caring

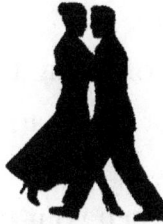

Marriage takes two to tango. Developing a marriage is like learning to dance with another person. Sometimes each partner steps on the toes of the other and trips. Time and effort are needed to develop harmony of movement. Both partners require emotional intelligence, the capacity to respectfully respond and care for the other while adjusting to the changing music of life. Emotional intelligence is expressed through empathy, sensitivity to others, and common sense to do the "right thing." It is another component of your internal GPS.

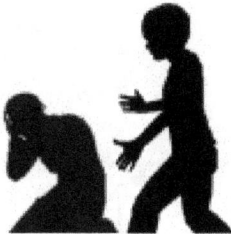

Empathy is a primary ability, skill and emotion that is developed. It is mentally and emotionally "standing in the shoes of another" by first focusing to shut out distractions so as "to understand [cognitive empathy] and share the feelings [affective empathy] of another".[85] It is transcending one's self to identify with the struggle of another. Low levels of empathy lead to cruelty.

Questions that can be asked to discern the extent to which empathy and caring for others is part of a marital candidate's character are:

- What experiences of caring for others have you had?
- Are you hard or easy to please? Please provide examples?
- What do you do when your parents, siblings or friends have had a hard day?
- How would you describe the way that you communicate with your parents, siblings, friends?
- What do you feel is the role of empathy in your future marriage? Please provide examples for how you have demonstrated empathy for your family members, for friends, for co-workers.

Spiritual Connection:
Motivation for Empathy and Compassion

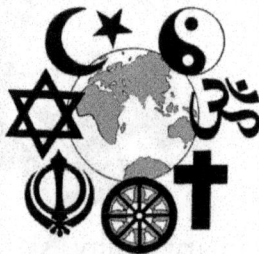

There must be a source of motivation to sustain unconditional commitment, empathy and kindness in marriage. Answers to the Indicator questions about an individual's "spiritual core" in Benchmark One can reveal what purposes they believe are worth living for that are greater than their self. They can indicate the level of their capacity for unconditional commitment to live life together with their mate in sickness and in health. They can reveal their capacity for empathy and compassion. Compassion is needed when one is unable or it is counterproductive to empathize with the emotions of one's mate. Spouses suffering from dementia and Alzheimer's disease, for example, may experience delusions, hallucinations and paranoia. It is difficult to empathize with those experiences. Compassion may be better suited, which is the desire to understand and to alleviate the suffering.

Willing and Able to Give and Receive

The ability to give and receive true love in one sense is simply about the willingness and ability to give and receive. Seligman distinguishes true love and intimacy from the Western notion of romance and sexual relationship, drawing attention to a common inability among men in Western culture to receive love.

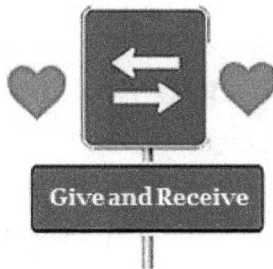

99

Men may care for others in admirable ways in terms of acts of unselfish generosity and empathy, but not allow themselves the same. For both male and female candidates it would be helpful to ask:

- Is it hard for you to open up to others?
- What subject do you find difficult to talk about?
- Do you find it difficult to receive encouragement and praise from others?

True love and true intimacy are reciprocal in nature. For each spouse to be emotionally, sexually and spiritually nourished in a marriage, they must have the capacity to communicate about and to reconcile differences in personality and frequency of desire for sexual relationships. It is part of the process of moving from self-centeredness to other-centeredness, from dependence to interdependence, from "me" to "we."

When men talk about sex and reference sex studies, how semen has hormones that benefit the woman partner, it is often from a male's perspective. When a husband has sex with his wife, he may think that it "counts" when only he has an orgasm. What about his wife? Becoming "as one" means that the husband makes efforts to assure his wife is also fulfilled...and better satisfied first in lovemaking.[86]

Capacity for Gratitude

Emotionally intelligent couples value their marriages by learning how to genuinely care for one another. They express care by cultivating their capacities for empathy, humility, gratitude and forgiveness. Communication skill building, such as empathic listening and assuring one's partner that they heard what was said, is also important. Skillful communication has its limits, though, as experienced relationship education trainers will tell you. It must be connected to experiencing gratitude--recognizing the priceless value of one's life partner and for their marriage. Marriage educator John Gottman laments that "[o]ne of the saddest reasons a marriage dies is that neither spouse recognizes its value until it is too late."[87]

A candidate's capacities for gratitude can be discovered by simply asking:

- What are you grateful for? Please explain.
- To whom are you grateful? Please explain.
- How do you express gratitude? Is it easy for you to express gratitude?
- How do you feel gratitude relates to marriage?

Forgiveness

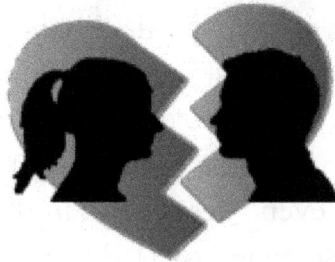

Forgiveness is a necessary part of turning toward one another in marriage rather than turning away when one feels hurt and wronged. Forgiveness as a virtue and as a psychological concept can be a little difficult to grasp and practice because different types of forgiveness apply to different situations and relationships. Generally speaking, though, psychologists "define forgiveness as a conscious, deliberate decision to release feelings of resentment and/or vengeance toward a person or group who has harmed you, regardless of whether they actually deserve your forgiveness."[88]

Forgiveness does not mean that one forgets the harm, condones or excuses the offense. Forgiveness is vital for basic mental health. People who forgive are healthier and happier than those who hold grudges and resentments. Forgiveness frees your mind of toxic anger so it does not control you; it enables healing and moving on in one's life. Forgiveness is a learned process, a disciplined practice, and therefore, requires time, support and intentional management of one's thoughts.

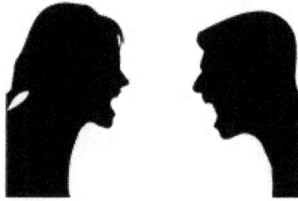

Growing up can be hard. Sibling rivalries and other family experiences can stir up angry feelings that one was treated unfairly. Negative childhood experiences, if not managed with forgiveness, can cause layers of resentment to fester, and even negatively impact one's marriage. Ideally, the discipline to forgive is developed from childhood. Questions like the following could be asked:

- How did you deal with conflicts with your siblings during childhood? Is it any different today?
- What do you do when someone has wronged you? Do you have an example?

- Is it hard for you to forgive others?
- Is there someone whom you have not been able to forgive?
- Have you ever been forgiven for something that you did wrong?

Intellectual Curiosity

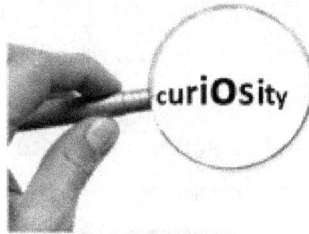

Few will dispute that spouses desire to engage in stimulating conversations with their beloved to feel *connected*. The persistent desire to know and learn about something, a skill, a place, an idea, or another person, especially one's spouse, is intellectual curiosity. It is not only important for personal growth, but also important for a couple's marital and sexual health—indeed, the mind/brain is a sexual organ. Ask marital candidates (potentials) about their objects of curiosity, their interests and their purposes underlying them, for instance, is it relaxation, self-improvement, or service to others?

- What things interest you beyond your current line of work or study?
- Do you have hobbies? What do you enjoying doing?
- What do you read? How regularly?

Creativity and the Arts

It is natural to think of one's self as being creative and desire to share one's life with someone who also desires to be creative. Like other abilities, the use of imagination to create new things must be well managed. Make sure that you clarify what a candidate means by being creative, especially if you or your potential spouse are very passionate about your art, particularly the performing or fine arts. The popular wisdom for serious artists is that "you must experience suffering to achieve true insight and inspiration." Some academics and heroin-addicted artists affirm that they must descend into the depths of darkness, anguish and pain to be creative.

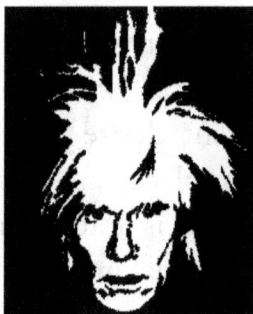

Pop culture admires the "tortured artist," who is explosive and self-destructive, and revolves in and out of drug rehabilitation. Troubled artists are elevated to be celebrity prophets, priests and priestesses, whose abuse of themselves, their romantic partners and children is excused by their celebrity.

Elizabeth Gilbert, author of *Eat, Pray, Love*, warns about those dark presumptions in her book *Big Magic*. Gilbert traces the mythology of "you must suffer to be authentically creative" to Western culture's heritage of Christian sacrifice and German Romanticism. In that context she advises, "Addiction does not make the artist." Indeed, true creativity does not spring from pathology and addiction. [89] Neuroscientist David Linden, at the John Hopkins University School of Medicine, agrees that alcoholics and drug addicts are not more creative because of their addiction. Dependence is not a source of creativity.[90]

Nonetheless, Gilbert's readers may not separate her warnings from her life course. Aspiring artists may think that they, too, must emulate her decisions and to divorce their spouses as a precondition to embark on a spiritual quest to India.

Very creative people who "think outside the box" may also think that "rules are meant to be broken," which can lead to a slippery slope of dishonesty. Creative people can use their creativity to justify very questionable behavior.

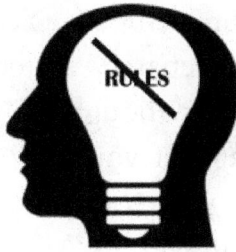

Consider how closely a potential mate connects their creativity with their personal disappointments, pain and suffering. Questions that might be asked are:

- What does it take to be really passionate and creative?
- How do you achieve authentic creativity?
- Which artists do you admire and why?
- What do you think about "tormented artists"?

- What does "rules are meant to be broken" mean to you?

Potential for Abuse

When it comes to marriage, forethought is better than afterthought. It is prudent to ask questions that individuals may be uneasy to talk about:

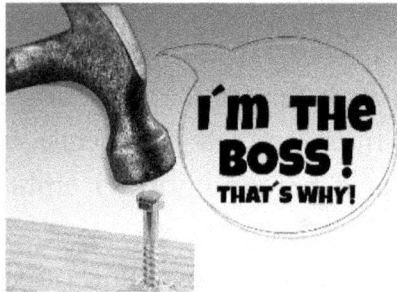

An individual may presume that they are suspected of committing abuse when asked those questions. Their responses can be very revealing. Observe whether they lose their composure or temper. You can preface your interviews with a prepared statement like "these are standard questions that thoughtful people consider when preparing for marriage. If you are offended by any of the questions, we ask for your forgiveness in advance. We hope that you can be patient with us."

- How is respect expressed in marriage?
- How is disrespect expressed in marriage?
- How could you cause harm to your spouse?
- Was there abuse in your family?
- Did you suffer abuse in your family? How did you respond?
- How do you feel about that?

- Were you bullied in school? How did you respond?

Our social bonds are transformative and can affect how long we live, how healthy we are, or how quickly we recover from an illness. Likewise, the person you marry can affect how long you live, how healthy you are, or how quickly you recover from an illness.

The Three Benchmarks are interrelated. That will be evident in the next and third Benchmark. Emotional and spiritual connection is also about social intimacy, and the ability to collaborate within the framework of institutions. Marriage, family and religious organizations are institutions which serve to catch you when you fall down and build you up to be your best.

CHAPTER 5

STEP 1: PREPARATION--
BENCHMARK THREE

"Interdependence is and ought to be as much the ideal of man as self-sufficiency. Man is a social being." --Mohandas Gandhi

Capacity to Collaborate Interdependently

The Compatibility Myth

Benchmark Three, the capacity to collaborate interdependently, is distinct from mere "compatibility" as it is popularly understood.

Compatibility is a buzz word deeply rooted within the popular psyche. It has broad acceptance as a basis of marriage and is often used synonymously for getting along well and having overlapping preferences and hobbies. Popular thinking presumes that it refers to a unique list of combined interests and personality traits essential for a couple to be happy without conflict. A couple either has that special mix or they do not. It is all or nothing. Current divorce rates at nearly 50 percent, however, suggest that our understanding of compatibility as the basis for marriage is either unreliable or does not present a complete picture of what a successful marriage requires.

The popular notion of compatibility for marriage is a myth. If lasting and nurturing interpersonal harmony is the real meaning of compatibility, then it is about more than whether the interests, hobbies and intellectual levels of two people are similar. Political preferences or affinities for particular types of music, TV and food, are factors that influence the everyday experience of marriage; however, they are not what holds a marriage together for a lifetime.

No Perfect Personality Fit Needed

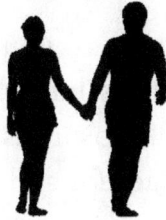

Neither is having a perfect fit of personality traits the key to a healthy marriage. Marriage researchers such as Gottman have observed that there is only a weak connection between failed marriages and couples with personality hang-ups and the ordinary type of fears or anxieties.

Gottman advises that the important thing is how a couple manages their personality differences. He warns against various myths that contribute to couples losing hope for their marriage. One is that personality weaknesses can ruin a marriage.

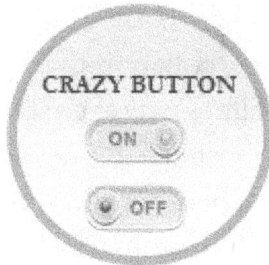

Gottman cautions, "We all have our crazy buttons – issues we're not totally rational about. But they don't necessarily interfere with marriage." After decades of research, he concludes that "the key to a happy marriage isn't having a 'normal' personality but finding someone with whom you mesh."[91] How well a couple manages their difficulties determines whether their marriage will thrive or die.

Be certain, though, that you identify any emotional triggers, anxieties or obsessions that you or your potential mate may have. Full disclosure is necessary for candidates to knowingly agree to accept and manage those conditions as a helpmate. Possible questions are:

- Do you have any "quirk" that you are working on that your future spouse might help you with?
- Does it sometimes get the best of you?
- How do you deal with it when it happens?

Appearances of Happiness Can Mask Terminal Problems

Gottman's research continues to be corroborated by other social science studies. For instance, psychologists Justin Lavner and Thomas Bradbury studied couples who had high levels of satisfaction during their first four years of marriage. Those that divorced during the next six years were those whose collaborative, communication and problem-solving abilities were unstable. They more easily argued and sharply criticized one another, did not listen well, and withdrew when conflicts arose.[92] Their behaviors were consistent with Gottman's "Four Horsemen," i.e., criticism, defensiveness, contempt, and stonewalling (withdrawal) that destroy marriages.[93] Thus, initial years of marital contentment may mask toxic problems that could lead to future divorce.

What will determine the health of your marriage is how well you and your spouse handle your difficulties--ordinary sources of conflict such as money, kids, sex, stress, in-laws, time, housework, as well as the extraordinary ones--and how well you can turn toward one another and positively connect emotionally during both good and bad times. It is imperative that couples travel in the same direction and grow together. Otherwise, they will drift apart under the daily stresses of marriage. If couples do not collaborate interdependently, then like two mismatched gears, they will grate against each other, grind to a halt and cease "working."

Binding Factors

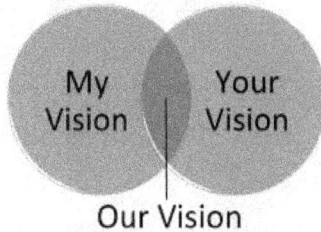

My Vision   Your Vision

Our Vision

As a practical matter, in marriage, long-lasting harmonious unity has more to do with a shared concept for the meaning of life, its purposes and priorities, a shared vision for the future and goals, and an agreement on the ways and means to those ends. Benchmarks One and Two address some of these fundamental issues.

Skillful Communication Helps

Couples can improve their ability to cooperate and reconcile the conflicting demands in marriage with interpersonal communication training. Such skill building is a major focus of the marriage education movement. Many businesses also include communication development as part of their management and employee training. Ask:

- Have you attended interpersonal communication training classes?
- If so, what did you learn from them?
- How have you applied lessons learned?

At the same time, skillful communication is not the complete answer to healthy marriages. Gottman concludes that it is a major misconception to believe that learning how to communicate with greater sensitivity will save your marriage. Couples who may be technically proficient with communication skills still divorce after many years of marriage.[94]

Communication is like plumbing in a house. While galvanized pipes may be replaced with more suitable copper tubing, if the water that travels through the plumbing is toxic, people will get sick drinking it. Criticism, defensiveness, contempt, and stonewalling are common forms of toxic communication that can harm a marriage. Therefore, the content of what is directly and indirectly expressed through skilled marital communication, not just the process of communication, is vital.

Compromise vs. Interdependence

Healthy marital collaboration is more than creating compromises between two strong, self-reliant and independent individuals who make concessions. It involves a higher level of mature, positive interaction.

Interdependence enables a couple to not only co-exist, but also to flourish.

Détente with Shallow Trust and Intimacy

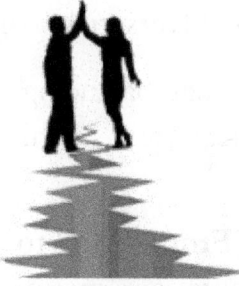

Compromise implies the settling of conflicts by each party making concessions — the loss of something by each. This no-win, no-lose arrangement resembles a tie and is not always satisfying. If a couple's approach to maintaining their relationship is to compromise (50/50), they may achieve a certain level of détente but not necessarily a deep level of trust and intimacy.

Some married couples stay in their marriage to maintain their status quo. They may see no promising alternative to their existing partner, may be constrained by fear of financial loss, or may fear compromising their children's well-being through a divorce.

Balancing

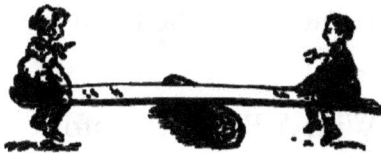

Consider the decision-making method of "balancing," which some people use to achieve work-life stability. It involves a process of weighing the pros and cons of competing interests. The Supreme Court uses it to decide the outcomes of two adversarial positions.

- Do you think that balancing is the best method to resolve conflicts and achieve satisfaction in a marriage?

From "Me" to "We"!

Interdependence is a superior method of decision-making that represents a change in motivation and behavior from "me" to "we," and engages elevated levels of creativity, empathy, and problem solving. It is the experience of synergy where 1 + 1 equals 3 or more and is the path to greater intimacy and "oneness." [95] Interdependence seeks a win-win result through what Covey calls "third alternative" solutions, arrived at through synergy and four paradigm shifts–"I See Myself, "I See You", "I Seek You Out," and "I Synergize With You."[96] When applied to marriage, it transcends conflict and is a more fulfilling experience. Covey explains it as:

"...in your heart you essentially say, 'My love for you is so great and our happiness is so entwined that I would not feel good if I got my way and you were unhappy—particularly when you feel so strongly about it."[97]

Win-Win, A Recent Historical Discovery

WIN- WIN

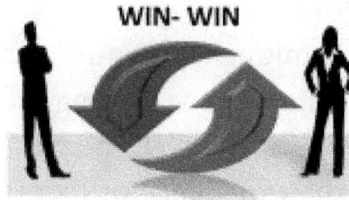

Interdependence is actually a very recent method of conflict resolution in history. It is both astonishing and tragic to learn that it took thousands of years for human beings to recognize an alternative to the adversarial system, which is inherently a competitive system whereby one party wins and the other loses. In the mid-twentieth century, psychologists Kurt Lewin and Morton Deutsch discovered that people could pursue a win-win solution if their *motivations focused on shared goals* and if they were willing to work together as partners instead of competitors to discover and implement a shared solution.[98] Motivation is key.

Real Compatibility = Interdependence

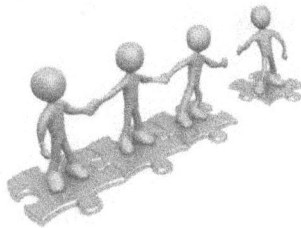

If compatibility is defined as the capacity for sustained cooperation that achieves high levels of synergy and creativity, then it is the result of interdependence, the ability to transition from *me* to *we*.

"We," a Shared Vision

True marital love and growth are about making unconditional commitments to further a common vision that achieves the highest well-being of one another and purposes beyond self-interest. Senge affirms that self-mastery leads to the experience of increasingly seeing one's connectedness with the world and a broader vision.[99] Thus, singles who are ready for marriage can better appreciate the value of interdependence and understand that their personal growth and fulfillment can be byproducts of marriage.

Self-Reliance

A couple may float into marriage on the wings of (false) romantic love; however, at some point those wings will not sustain the realities of living together. Self-reliance and independence are building blocks toward interdependence. Ask questions about a candidate's view of self-reliance:

- How have you demonstrated self-reliance?

- Have you lived away from home and been financially responsible for your own affairs?

- What were the reasons behind ending your employment at your past job(s)?

- What did you learn from those experiences?

- Do you currently have a paying job?

- Do you/will you have student loans?

- When was the last time you checked your credit rating?

- Do you have employment experience? What was your longest period of employment at any one place?

Career Plans

Decades of stagnating and declining wages and growing income inequality are forcing both husbands and wives to earn an income to maintain a family. It is important to inquire about an individual's short and long-term career plans and aspirations:

- What is your plan for career development?
- What are you doing to further that plan?

Work First vs. Family First

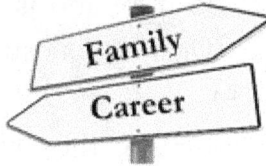

Making a living is hard and can take its toll on marriages. The US is a country with a "work first" culture of dual-income couples, who are working increasingly more hours and stressing how to provide for their families, to rear their children, and to bring their family and work into a "balance." CNN journalist and father Josh Levs' reports his painful personal work and family experiences, which led him to document them in his book *All In: How Our Work-First Culture Fails Dads, Families, and Businesses--And How We Can Fix It Together*. He explains how workplace environments and wages in the past 50 years have not kept pace with changes in the needs and roles of men and women in the family.[100]

Adding to the difficulty of giving one's family the attention that it needs are pop culture's negative stereotyping of fathers as being uninvolved, lazy and incompetent caregivers, of mothers as supermoms who can do it all, and that divorce is normal.

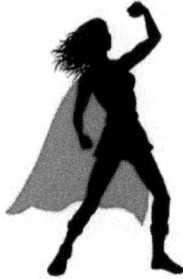

Super Mom

Can women *really* do it all and is divorce *really* normal? One could ask the following questions about roles in a family:

- Do you think you have the ability to be a husband (wife)? Please explain why.
- What do you feel are the roles of a husband and wife in a family?
- Do you think you have the ability to be a father/mother? Please explain why.
- What are the roles of a father and a mother in a family?
- Can or should mothers be "supermoms?" Can they do it all?
- What does a father contribute to his son's life? His daughter's life?
- What does a mother contribute to her son's life? Her daughter's life?

Married Single vs. Married Married

As many married couples do, they confuse independence and self-reliance such that they think and act as "married singles," giving priority to career, self-development, individual hobbies, and retaining separate bank accounts, rather than prioritizing their marriage. Their focus on "me" rather than on "we" inclines them to drift apart.

If, on the other hand, couples prioritize their decisions around "we"—their marriage, then their foundation of commitment, intimacy and collaboration is strengthened as a "married-married" couple. Consider asking:

- How much time do you feel you need in your schedule for pursuing professional or personal development, or for enjoying individual interests and hobbies?
- Do you plan to have separate bank accounts when you start off your marriage?
- Do you think that your lifestyle will change once you are married? How so?

Being Complementary: A Helpmate On the Road to "We"

When a couple marry, they join as two imperfect and uniquely different individuals committed (hopefully) to be the helpmate of one another during the romantic and heroic life journey of becoming the best that each can be.

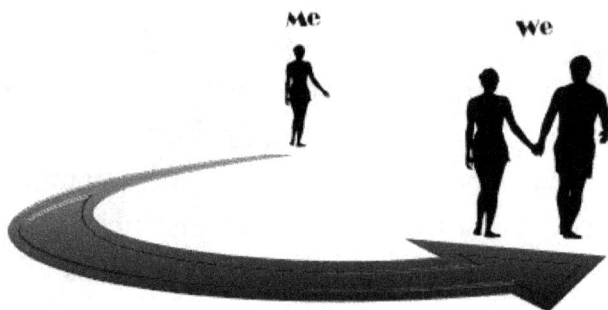

One of the unconditional commitments mentioned earlier is to the highest well-being of one's spouse. This recognizes that no one enters marriage as a perfectly formed person. While pre-marriage education and interpersonal skill building can equip a couple with important social skills for marriage, being each other's helpmate to heal and enrich one another's soul (soulmate) requires knowledge of what to help and how to help.

There is no perfect matching set of personality traits for a couple to be compatible. If individuals have the attitudes and skills to positively adjust within an ordinary range of personality differences, they can learn to synergize and deal with their differences, and to become happy through interdependence. Birds of a feather may flock together but birds can be different and complementary.

It is important to consider complementary personality qualities in candidates which would enable them to be better together than alone. This does not refer simply to opposites, such as one spouse being generally strong and the other generally weak. The strengths of one spouse can support and/or offset a weakness or imbalance of the other to become balanced and whole.

Can Be Better Together

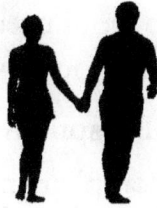

Couples who have personality differences can learn to be better together. While learning to negotiate differences may initially need more effort as a couple, these differences can help a couple become more effective as a team. For instance, one partner who is more social and the other more detail-oriented can be complementary. The wife may be more social and better at calling guests and getting the cooperation of family, friends, or colleagues for an event, while the husband may prefer and be more effective at planning and implementing the event. Or vice versa. Through this division of tasks, a husband and wife can help one another get things done with reduced stress and a satisfying sense of partnership.

One spouse may be more artistic and the other more practical. One may be more extroverted and the other more introverted. One may be more serious and the other more light-hearted. Over the course of a lifetime, different personalities may also have more interesting conversations than those who are similar in personality.

Complementing one another requires the capacity for humility, empathy, patience and forgiveness. Therefore, identify the complementary traits in potential mates that may benefit from being counterbalanced or enhanced. Here is an important question to ask:

- What qualities do you need in an ideal spouse to become the best that you can be?

Character vs. Personality--Easy to Confuse

When identifying complementary traits in a potential spouse, it is important to distinguish between character and personality. It is easy to confuse them because we presume the best in people whose personalities we like. If a person is friendly and attractive, we may presume that they are trustworthy, kind and moral.

Character refers to the pattern of a person's moral/ethical behaviors, which are motivated and shaped by beliefs learned during a lifetime. Those character traits may be good or bad and expressed through thoughts, words, and behaviors. Commonly referenced positive and negative character traits are: honest and dishonest, kind and mean, loyal and disloyal, courteous and impolite, friendly and unfriendly, hard-working and lazy, humble and arrogant, respectful and rude, brave and cowardly. In common speech "a person of character" is presumed to have good character, which is a compliment.

Personality, on the other hand, is unique to each person and commonly assumed to be what we were born with. It includes the way you see the world, think, and make decisions.

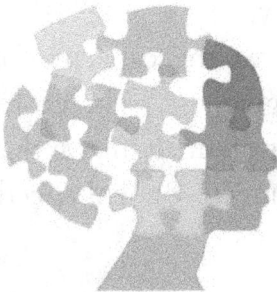

People can immediately and generally categorize personality types into reserved introverts or bubbly extroverts, sensitive and thin-skinned or insensitive and thick-skinned, open and adventurous or closed and cautious, dominant or passive.

Character is much more difficult to identify than personality, which is easier to read. Therefore, a multi-layered approach to assessing readiness for marriage is prudent.

Cross-Referencing

By cross-referencing candidates' opinions with their biographies, autobiographies, and interviews, gradually a composite or mental picture of their personality traits materializes. There are various personality tests that can also provide insight, from those developed by Hippocrates in 400 B.C. [101] to Katharine Cook Briggs/Isabel Briggs Myers (Myers-Briggs Type Indicator) [102] and Peter Urs Bender. [103] The Flagpage is also useful. [104] Research the different ways that psychologists have categorized personality types and glean from them what is useful.

Good Character Must Manage Personality

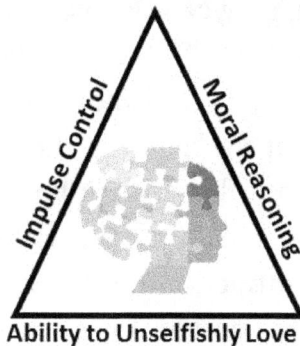

A key factor to remember is that each personality trait has a certain strength and can beome a weakness if not well managed by good character. Someone who is analytical and disciplined in nature could become overly perfectionistic and demanding. A person who is passionate, decisive and driven could become uncooperative and overbearing. Someone who is patient and supportive could lack assertiveness when needed. The charming and charismatic person could become narcissistic.

Strengths can become weaknesses when under a lot of stress. For example, as pressure builds, the drive to achieve excellence and success may lead one to lose adaptability. There are people who are very nurturing and desire to take care of others, who invest themselves to such an extent in others that they deplete their mental and emotional gas tanks and become exhausted. The organized person can become controlling and rigid and the spontaneous person can become irresponsible.

Fatal Attractions: First Impressions

First impressions, triggered by the hormonal chemistry of passionate (false) romantic love can be strongly positive or negative; in fact, they can be overwhelming.

Have you heard of "fatal attraction?" No, we don't mean the 1987 psychological movie thriller *Fatal Attraction*. We are talking about the fact that the very same personality qualities that romantically attract two people can contribute to destroying their relationship. "Exciting and different" are common fatal attraction characteristics.[105] Attraction to charming, confident, and funny narcissistic people is also common. Sociology professor Diane Felmlee coined the term "fatal attraction" over two decades ago in her innovative research to describe those behaviors.

A decade after Felmlee's initial research, psychotherapist Ayala Malach Pines advanced that Felmlee's fatal attraction phenomenon was far more common than her data indicated: "In virtually every case of the hundreds with whom I have worked in couple therapy and in couple groups, if the relationship was based on romantic love, it was possible to find a connection between the traits that attracted the couple to each other and the traits that later became the focus of their problems."[106]

Knowledge of the fatal attraction phenomenon can assist in selecting a lifelong mate.

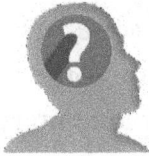

Reflect and ask yourself,
- How might the personality quality of this person become excessive and a fatal attraction?

Marriage partners help one another to maintain emotional, mental, and spiritual balance and resilience. That comes with interdependence, when a couple share a common set of principles while valuing one another's differences in personality, interests, abilities, strengths and weaknesses.

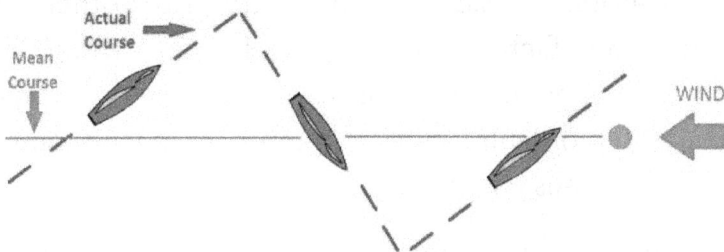

A fitting metaphor is a plane or boat "tacking," which means making zigzagging adjustments to cross winds to stay on course to its destination. As cross winds push a plane or boat off course, a marriage partner may be pushed off balance by stress and disappointments. They need compensating support to stay on a healthy life course.

Not a Scorecard

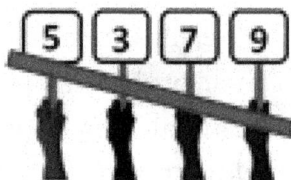

Everyone has strengths and weaknesses. There is a common tendency to feel accused if someone observes that you have a weakness or are out of balance in some way. When we consider how two people are complementary, it is not a scorecard exercise to determine who has more points than the other or to assure that each has the same number of weak or imbalanced areas as the other. In addition, it is important to consider that relative weaknesses, imbalances and strengths often change during the course of a marriage.

If a husband and wife are to become genuine helpmates and collaborators, each must be aware of the other's needs. During the fact-finding stage of the 7-Step Family Approach, it would be helpful to ask each candidate to review the biography, autobiography, interviews, and other personality assessments of the other and ask:

- What qualities does he/she need in an ideal spouse to be the best that he/she can be?

If a couple is to form a nurturing partnership, they must have a basic understanding of the nature, personality, character, hopes, dreams and fears, strengths and weaknesses of the other. This includes an understanding of one another's families.

Candidate's Family History

It is reasonable to say that one's birth family experience shapes to a great extent, for good or ill, how one cooperates and resolves disagreements and conflicts in one's marriage. Questions to ask are:

- How did your parents address conflict in your home?
- How did you address disagreements with your parents?
- How did you address disagreements with your siblings (or extended family/close family friends, if no siblings)?
- How did your family resolve disagreements?
- Will the way you approach cooperation and resolving disagreements in your marriage be different from your family experience? If so, why and how?

Take care to evaluate how well the potential spouse cooperates with their parents during the 7-Step Family Approach.

If candidates have had low-trust relationships with their parents, there is a good chance their low-trust behaviors may extend to the in-laws and compromise their marriages. Present this scenario to a potential candidate: Joann complains to her husband Don, "Your mother shows no respect for me, yet she expects me to respect her. If you don't make her respect me, I won't allow our kids to see her." Consider:

- If you are single considering a person like Joann, ask yourself, "Could I manage the potential conflicts? How would I do it?"

It has been said before, marriage between two people is also a marriage between their two families. As a certain range of conflicts are normal in marriage, so are conflicts with in-laws. There will be potential relational conflicts in just about any human organization. Every family has some issues: sometimes there is a family member--a brother, sister, a parent, brother-in-law, sister-in-law--who is very troubled and sends ripples of instability that impact the entire extended family. The marriage vow of "in sickness and in health" extends to your spouse's family. Questions to consider asking are:

- Do you have a family member who is really hard to get along with? Why?

- Are you willing to accept "the full package" of family issues that comes with the potential spouse? Do you know what they are?

- How would you handle future conflicts with your future in-laws? How would you prefer that your future spouse handles future conflicts with your direct family members?

CHAPTER 6

STEP 2: IDENTIFYING CANDIDATES & CREATING A FRAMEWORK FOR EXPLORATORY DISCUSSIONS

When people explore the possibilities of marriage, in both Western-style and arranged marriage traditions, they often have presumptions or unrealistic expectations that lead to regrettable missteps.

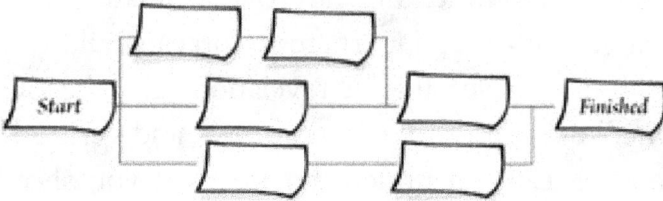

Make a Plan

When preparing for marriage, like preparing for any journey, it is prudent to plan and anticipate the various needs along the way. This chapter provides a method of identifying and screening potential marriage candidates and negotiating with parents a safe and smart framework for exploratory discussions and a measured process that could potentially lead to marriage.

Be Mr./Ms. Right to Find Mr./Ms. Right

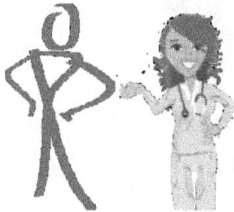

129

At this point you may be asking, "Where or how do we find suitable candidates for marriage whom to consider?" Our advice is that if you are single and looking for Mr. Right or Ms. Right, first assure that you are a Mr. Right or Ms. Right. Be the person of integrity, caring and love that you desire. You will more likely attract (law of attraction) a Mr. Right or Ms. Right. For those religiously inclined, you will be better attuned to understand and receive God's guidance to meet Mr. Right or Ms. Right.

At the same time, do not overestimate what God, Cupid, angels or other supernatural forces would or should do, and if you have sudden revelations that he or she is "the One," question those assumptions and verify them by other means. Do not underestimate what you should and can do, nor overestimate it, like assuming you have clairvoyance, telepathy, or a fortune-telling crystal ball for matchmaking.

If you are single, put into writing who you think you are and why you are ready for marriage--write a short autobiography of yourself.

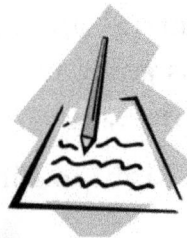

If you are the parents of a single son or daughter desiring marriage, become students of marriage and family, and make the effort to explain in writing who your daughter or your son is and why she or he is ready for marriage--write a short biography of them.

Then share and discuss your writings with one another, get on the same page, and plan how to walk together through *A Better Way To Marry*. Get marriage right from the start.

Looking for Love in the Right Places

Millions of single adults daily use a variety of matchmaking websites. The question is, though, "Are they looking for love in all the right or wrong places?" Put your mind and efforts in the right place. If you use an online website, be aware of the many hazards that are often there.

Most People Find Their Match Offline

Even though millions of Americans are using online dating websites, a 2016 Pew Research Center study found that only "5% of Americans who are in a marriage or committed relationship say they met their significant other online."[107]

Think...Family First!

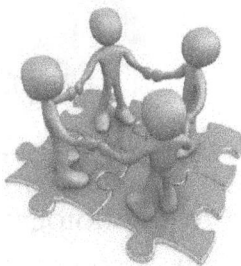

If you are single, form a supportive family team for the search--ideally with your parents as your greatest supporters and partners, and for all the many reasons that we have explained. You might include as part of your team other family members who care for you and can serve as a sounding board and provide you with recommendations. Search through your family networks.

Three Benchmark Analysis

The previously described Three Benchmarks and their Indicator questions can serve as the basis of a written "Three Benchmark Analysis" to identify and evaluate yourself (if you are seeking a spouse), your son or daughter, and potential marriage candidates who can be considered for further exploratory discussions. In other words, use the same yardstick to evaluate the individuals being considered as marital partners. Since there are over 200 Indicator questions, select 5 to 10 "big picture" Indicator questions, or as many that are helpful, for each of the Three Benchmarks.

A Better Way To Marry is about predicting future behavior in a potential marriage. A new prediction method called "coarse graining" can be learned from several fields such as physics, meteorology, biology and medicine.

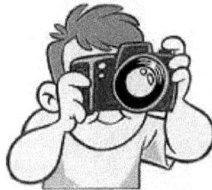

Originally derived from photography, course graining is a method of looking at a complex, detailed structure or system that focuses on an element within it, until you can see a rough outline of it, sufficient to generally understand what it is and its behavior. Meteorologists can look at the shape (the coarse-grain element) of clouds to forecast weather. Applied to searching for a lifelong mate, there is more to comprehend beyond quick first visual impressions when looking at a person's profile picture. There is much more beneath the surface to discover and it comes in layers. More focused effort is required.

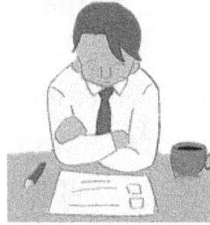

Everyone in the family team is advised to exercise due diligence when identifying anyone as a potential marriage partner, who we will call a "candidate." Also seek consensus among the family team's recommendations by using the same Indicator questions and sources to answer the questions. That would include but not be limited to each family team member reviewing a potential candidate's website profile, social media entries, and conducting discreet discussions with people who know the potential candidate.

Apply the same yardstick of Indicator questions for each candidate. Probably the content and depth of each potential candidate's profile descriptions will vary, and a potential may not reveal anything that could answer some of your questions. Nevertheless, do the best that you can with what is before you.

Copy and Paste It

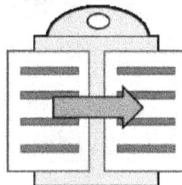

Under each marital readiness Indicator question, *copy exactly* what each candidate wrote in their profile (or other sources, e.g., Facebook) that answers your Indicator questions and *paste* it under the corresponding questions. After completing your list of Indicator questions with the candidate's answers, you can then evaluate what you think all the combined answers suggest about the potential candidate. This will help to maintain focus and objectivity.

If it is difficult to make distinctions between the potential candidates, try this. Create a spreadsheet for each candidate profile. Then, based on the written evaluations of each profile, provide a number from 1 to 10 with 10 being the highest that represents the *quality* of the response for each indicator answered by the candidate. For instance, give a numerical value (1 to 10) for each purpose-centered reason that would motivate a candidate to make unconditional commitments (Benchmark One) in marriage. It might be religious, ethical, family, other in nature. For each Indicator in Benchmark Two, such as empathy, humility, gratitude, give a numerical value (1 to 10).

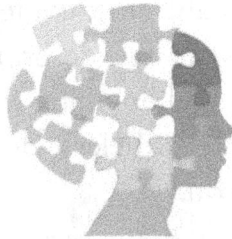

Like focusing the lens of a camera, layer upon layer of questions and answers can cause the image of the person's character and personality to come into focus. The layers are based upon what each individual has written or said, and what others have written or said about the individual. They form a baseline of knowledge that can be later verified.

Yes, it can be a challenging process looking at the profiles and pictures of several people. How do you know whether a person would make a good husband or wife? Since we are talking about a preliminary way of understanding someone, you won't know with confidence until you go through an additional verification process by evaluating further writings, discussions and experiences with a particular candidate. Some individuals may write what they think others want to see.

Identify the Top Three

Reflect, meditate, pray. Do whatever helps you focus and meaningfully rank the top three. Be cautiously optimistic while emotionally detached from the expectation that one of them will become your spouse. Do not become captive to the myth of the one-and-only soulmate. Choose one with whom to explore possibilities. The purpose of initiating a meeting with a potential candidate is not for casual dating. A recommended candidate is someone who has been seriously reviewed for their marriage potential. Therefore, they are not recommended exclusively on appearance or because they "look hot." If he or she does not materialize into an engagement, go to the next one on your list. Be patient.

Expand Three Benchmark Analysis
Thru the 7-Steps

The initial Three Benchmark Analysis provides an initial knowledge base to build upon as you progress through each step of the Family Approach process. More questions will likely be added to expand and verify your understanding of the inner life and character of the candidate considered for marriage.

Initial Contact

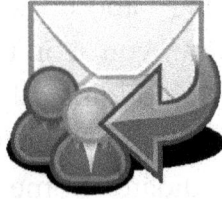

If you are the parent or trusted advisor of a single adult, exercise courtesy when initially contacting the parent or trusted advisor of a candidate you have identified. Be respectful and diplomatic. Take time to craft and send an introductory letter or e-mail. It is better than an abrupt phone call because the letter or e-mail creates some space for the other party to thoughtfully consider your comments and request. Express awareness and respect for the other candidate's bio profile and admirable qualities, and that you genuinely think your son/daughter could complement them. Invite the parent or trusted advisor to review your son's/daughter's profile and mention some of their admirable qualities. Assure that there is a way that your candidate's profile is accessible. Send it via e-mail or snail mail.

Prevent Heartbreak--Guidelines

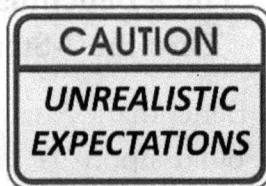

When people explore the possibilities of marriage, in both Western-style and Eastern, arranged-marriage traditions, they often have assumptions and unrealistic expectations that lead to regrettable missteps. If precautions are not taken, unspoken expectations, driven by the blind passion of (false) romantic love, or by conventions of one's social/ethnic/religious group, can lead to uninformed and unreflective decisions to rush into intimate relationships, and even to marry. Marriages often fail before they begin. Well thought out and mutually agreed upon guidelines serve as a safety net for respectful and meaningful discussions.

Premature Relationships in Western and Eastern Societies

In Western cultures, when a male and female experience physical attraction and start dating, they may regard themselves as boyfriend and girlfriend. If they are among almost 60 percent of "Middle Americans" who are young adults and high school graduates but not college graduates, it is likely that they will move in together without marrying. They have sex because that is what they see as normalized behavior in society. As boyfriend and girlfriend, they may say to each other, "I love you."

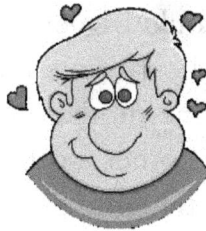

But what would their words really mean? Would they mean the type of love that would sustain a lifetime together in marriage? In the merry-go-round of hooking up and breaking up, 44 percent of Middle Americans will have babies, but will not marry.[108]

Amber and David Lapp, researchers at the Institute for American Values, tell the story of how Seth and Stephanie view marriage and say "I love you." Seth, a twenty-three-year old boyfriend of twenty-five-year old Stephanie, an unmarried mother of two, doubts that those "I love you" words and the way they started their relationship would stand the test of time. Their relationship began as a "spontaneous sexual encounter at a party that got too crazy, only days after breaking up with a girl whom he had hoped to marry."[109]

Pressure to Marry

Convention and tradition in Eastern societies have also been seen to propel people into premature relationships. In traditional, tribal Afghan culture, when parents explore the possibilities of marriage for their sons and daughters, they begin with discussions. In some tribal customs, when parents confirm the agreement of their son and daughter to marry, the mother of the girl gives a scarf to the boy's mother. If the scarf is not accepted, it is considered a grave offense. An offense could trigger violent tribal retaliation.

What if, before the parents sit down to discuss and explore possibilities, the mother of the young lady was to extend the scarf to the other mother? She could manipulate the power of rituals, tradition and honor codes to force a marriage. What a dilemma!

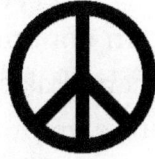

During the 1960s in Afghanistan and prior to the Soviet invasion in 1979, Kabul and other big cities were very cosmopolitan. Young, educated elites recognized the abuses and excesses in traditional arranged marriages in their country. Influenced by Westerners and their counterculture movement that was cascading across the world, young privileged Afghan men and women, criticized the tradition of arranged marriage and sought to be modern by falling in love as the basis for choosing their spouse. Living within a culture deeply rooted in tradition and an honor-shame code, many carefully masked their efforts to form their Western (false) romantic love marriages to save appearances and the honor of their families. Many of those who formed their marriages that way and were able to escape to Western countries during the civil war following the withdrawal of the Soviet Union in 1989, ended up trapped in loveless marriages when their passions of falling in love predictably faded away.

Globalization of Falling in Love

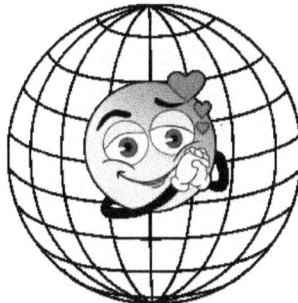

Today a similar pattern continues for young, single men and women from Afghan, Pakistani, Philippine, Korean, Vietnamese and other immigrant communities living in the US and Europe who seek to be like their Western friends by following more Western practices related to dating and marriage. Many fall in love and attempt to get their parents' approval either with their tears or with demands.

Nominated for three Academy Awards in 2016, *Brooklyn* tells the romantic love story of a young Irish girl, Eilis, who immigrated to Brooklyn, New York City. Eilis falls in love with a young Italian man, Tony. However, Tony fears that Eilis will not return to him when she is called back to Ireland after her sister's sudden death. Seeking to assure her return, Tony pressures Eilis to secretly marry him and to have sex with him a few hours before her ship departs for Ireland, to seal the deal. Not knowing whether the couple lived a happily-ever-after Hollywood marriage, one could argue that Tony unfairly manipulates Eilis.

Whether from Western culture or traditional Eastern cultures, safety nets are needed to prevent single adults from being pushed into ill-fated intimate relationships by intoxicating but illusory chemistry, loneliness, convention, or force of tradition.

Not Enough Information

Young singles often want to quickly start talking with another desirable single, especially if one or both impetuously think the other is their soulmate. Their parents may also think that falling in love is the natural thing to do. If they are over 18 years old, they probably regard themselves as legal adults, and also emotional adults. Why?

Simply because it is presumed to be self-evident, that any legal adult automatically knows whether someone is a suitable lifetime marriage partner and knows how to effectively communicate. It is just a matter of chemistry and, if you are in love, you will just know how.

Straight-up Bozos

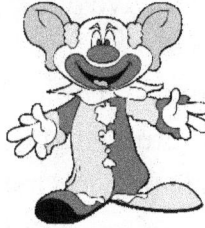

Do single, legal adults really know how to effectively communicate when seeking a spouse? Are they socialized to be emotional adults who act with respect? The Aziz Ansari and Eric Klinenberg study of online dating concludes "that most dudes out there are straight-up bozos" in their first texts to women.[110] Consider, too, that there is a tragically high rate of dating violence and sexual abuse.

Common Misconceptions

What are some of the common misconceptions that could prevent genuine communication between two single adults that would verify whether they are, in fact, a good match for marriage?

One could wrongly presume that each has enough information to know what is going on between them. If they are not on the same page or in the same ballpark of understanding, how can they begin to deeply share and examine their beliefs, perceptions, and feelings about the fundamentals of life?

Another misconception could involve incorrectly presuming that each understands what the other thinks or feels is the purpose of their communication. Even if they think the purpose is determining whether they are a good match, ready for marriage, compatible and complementary or the like, each could have very different ideas of what that means.

A third misconception could be that each individual understands their mutual expectations for disclosing "personal" information that is vital to a marriage decision, the number and types of questions to ask, procedures to follow such as how to respectfully end the discussions if one party so chooses, and more.

Guidelines Agreement

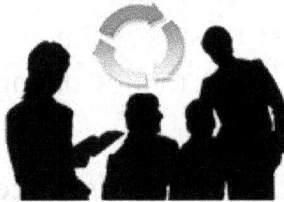

Make a plan for how you will communicate with a candidate and their family that anticipates that they may have different ideas about how to explore marital possibilities. It can minimize or prevent misunderstandings.

Exchange Ideas for Exploratory Discussions

As a matter of prudence and diplomacy, respectfully suggest that both parties begin by exchanging their ideas for exploratory discussions. Assure that all parties understand the reasons for the discussions and the value for whatever they agree upon. Passively acquiescing to "whatever" or "we'll see what happens with whatever" can lead to painful disappointments. The following are examples of two purposes for exploratory discussions:

- Facilitate meaningful discovery as to whether the candidates are ready for marriage, compatible/interdependent, complementary, and could commit to a shared life vision;
- Create a safe environment that benefits all parties to experience meaningful discovery and to make informed decisions.

Suggested Guidelines

Consider the following guidelines to further these purposes:

1. *Discussions are exclusive between the two candidates and their families.* During the discussions, if others contact you to consider their candidate, inform them that you are currently in discussions with another family/candidate.

2. *All parties agree that merely entering into discussions does not guarantee an eventual engagement.* On the other hand, all parties agree to enter into discussions without being predisposed to reject the other candidate. Humans are not commodities. Candidates agree to begin with an open mind and to participate in honest dialogue and mutual discovery. If one's heart is not in the right place and is deeply conflicted with the idea of marriage or with marrying this particular candidate, do not enter into discussions. If an engagement does

not result after initiating discussions, the goal is that all parties would have benefited by greater self-awareness and mutual awareness and respect.

3. *Be virtue centered rather than fantasy centered.* Look for the qualities of character that make for a caring and reliable life partner. Do not compare one another with an unattainable person, or a fantasy candidate, nor be fixated on preconceived notions of there being only one specific "my type" of person for marriage. Couples do not enter marriage as perfectly formed soulmates. The temporary euphoria and declarations of falling in love are neither the genuine gold standards nor self-evident bases to sustain a marriage. True love is learned and *couples become soulmates.*

A safe, reliable way to marry is not a stress-free experience. It is a very emotional process where patience, restraint and steadiness are needed. It is common to feel anxious or fearful of rejection, of being hurt, of making the "wrong" decision. Although those emotions are real and understandable, they must still be managed.

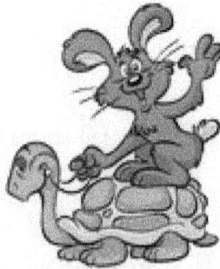

4. *Slower is better, safer and faster. Seek first to understand.* Personality can be quickly recognized. However, it is

different from character, the predictor of future behavior. Time and experience are required to reveal and verify one's character.

5. *Disclose all material facts to enable informed decisions.*

   a. At the appropriate times, parents agree to exchange and discuss the written biographies of their son/daughter—a brief history and description of their personality and character, and reasons why they think their son/daughter is ready for marriage.

   b. Candidates agree to exchange and discuss their autobiographies--written self-descriptions of who they are, their history, personality and character, and reasons why they are ready for marriage.

   c. In writing, either before or during discussions, the parties agree to disclose whether the candidate has had a dating history, sexual relations with others, and any sexually transmitted diseases (STDs) or HIV. Make it simple by providing a document signed by a qualified medical professional disclosing the results of HIV/STD blood tests. Disclose whether the candidate has a personal or family history of mental or physical illnesses or addictions, substance abuse, or a criminal record.

   d. Commitment to the highest well-being of one's spouse and forgiveness are needed for a marriage to survive and thrive. To be a helpmate, a spouse must know what to help. After the biographies, autobiographies and interviews have been completed, each candidate agrees to write and

145

explain, in their opinion, the qualities in an ideal spouse the other candidate needs to be the best that they can be.

6. *Respect.* Questions and responses by each party are to be respected, which includes replying in a timely manner (within three days is suggested) to a question or a request through any form of communication, such as phone calls, e-mails, and letters. This does not mean that you must agree with all requests or opinions. There can be misunderstandings due to cultural or personality differences, or presumptions such as how and when candidates should talk with one another. Any party can decline to answer a question. All parties, though, agree to clearly convey that decision to the others. Lack of timely communication can create misunderstandings.

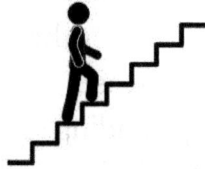

7. *Step-by-step.* After each step or conversation, ask, "What are your thoughts about next steps?" Do not presume that the other party can read your mind or "should know." *If there is no full agreement by all parties to go to the next defined step,* then all parties agree in advance to respectfully conclude discussions and not condemn the other. Then hopefully this is regarded as a learning experience and a stepping stone toward the future. This measured approach encourages a meeting of the minds, friendship, and respect.

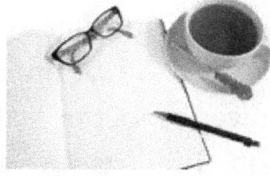

8. *Write Evaluations.* If, and once all parties (parents and candidates) arrive at this step and have had all their questions answered to their satisfaction, then each set of parents agrees to write an evaluation explaining whether or not and why they recommend their son/daughter to consider courtship with the other candidate. They agree to explain whether, in their opinion, the other candidate appears to have the potential to be a suitable spouse—i.e., is ready for marriage, compatible, complementary, can be interdependent.

The male and female candidates also agree in advance to, likewise at this stage, provide a written assessment of one another. The goals of these efforts are to provide meaningful reflection, an informed choice, and consensus building.

(Approximately three to six weeks may be involved for the above steps, and longer, if all parties agree that it is needed.)

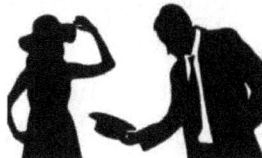

9. *Whether to Meet.* The candidates then decide whether to directly explore the possibilities of marriage with one another, in other words, courtship.

10. *Courtship.* If the candidates agree to personally discuss the possibilities of an engagement, they will follow a "slower is better" approach to personal communication. Importantly, agreeing to talk does not guarantee an engagement.

11. *Pre-Engagement Verification.* If during courtship, the candidates express a desire to be engaged, all parties (candidates and their parents) agree as two families to *mutually ask and answer questions* to verify that the couple is making a fully informed decision: for instance, questions such as "What are the reasons that you want to marry?", "How are you similar and different?", "What do you envision for your life together during the next 3 to 5 years?", "What challenges will you face?"

Is This Too Much to Ask?

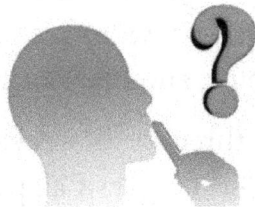

Consider what could happen if any of the above guidelines were not followed: if you did not enter into discussions with an open mind, did not screen out unrealistic expectations or manage your emotions, did not respect one another, or did not disclose all material facts. The purpose of these guidelines is to promote safety, mutual respect, meaningful discovery and informed decisions. Are those steps worth the effort? Do they seem too businesslike and not *romantic* enough? If it is you who is seeking a lifelong mate, ask yourself whether it is worth the effort.

Easier Said Than Done

While all parties may agree that merely entering into discussions would not guarantee that a "match" or that an engagement would occur, it is difficult to escape the inevitable hopes and fears that accompany such an important discussion. There is the hope that their candidate might be their future spouse, as well as fears of rejection and/or fear of making a wrong decision. The longer the process of fact-finding and courtship, the greater can be the frustration and disappointment when there is no resulting engagement.

Nevertheless, sufficient time, patience and emotional discipline are needed to make an informed decision for arguably the most important one in life--selection of a lifelong mate. If you have determined that this person is actually in your ballpark of possibility to be your lifelong partner, is it not worth the time and effort?

Naïve Independence vs. Interdependence

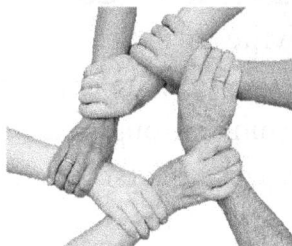

Some young adults may think that the involvement of their parents in the mate selection process makes them less than independent adults. On the contrary, just like a high degree of maturity is required for a couple to collaborate interdependently in marriage, young single adults and their parents are challenged to exercise a higher degree of maturity than naïve independence through this collaborative *Family Approach*. Certainly, every single adult should make the final decision regarding when and whom to marry. At the same time, for their marriage decision to be meaningful, it must be informed and based on wisdom and good judgment, which recognizes that the selection of a mate and formation of a marriage are not just between two people. Legally, emotionally and spiritually, marriage is between two families. Today, interdependence within and between families is even more important.

A Litmus Test

The willingness to provide full disclosure through the exchange of biographies and autobiographies and to discuss them is a litmus test.

Clear reflective writing may not be easy for many young adults and their parents. It is not a common practice in our computer-driven world where writing has become increasingly abbreviated through e-mails, texting and tweeting. For decades, most US schools have not taught students how to write analytically beyond essay questions that ask, "How do you feel?" People have lots to say, but it requires effort to think through and to express their ideas in writing so others can understand them.

If single males and females are unwilling to explain in writing who they are and why they are prepared for marriage, that could indicate a lack of seriousness, that they have something to hide, or that they do not think they need to prove their worthiness for marriage to another.

A single adult may sometimes think that they fully understand all of the knowledge that their parents possess when it comes to relationships or may think that there isn't much they can learn from their parents or other adults about marriage. A lack of humility compromises their capacity to be a "qualified" bachelor or bachelorette.

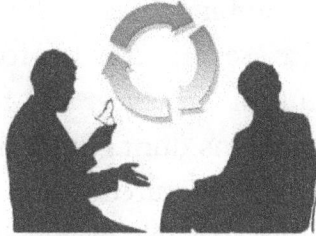

Sharing one's thoughts about life, love, marriage and family requires effort and humility. It is understandable to feel nervous when disclosing deeply personal information. Nonetheless, making good-faith efforts to explain who you are can serve as a starting point and basis for future in-person discussions. What is not expressed in a biography or autobiography, can later be addressed through follow-up Indicator questions.

CHAPTER 7

STEPS 3, 4, 5:
FACT-FINDING TO PRE-COURTSHIP

Marriage is a huge, life-changing commitment that requires coherent decisions based on realistic expectations. However authoritative you may think intuition, a revelation, a spark or an attraction is to justify a marriage decision, it must still be verified.

This chapter combines three *Family Approach* steps, which may require several weeks for the exchange of biographies and autobiographies, and for the discussion of many Indicator questions during interviews. Be patient. Let time be your friend. Measured steps of fact-finding can provide opportunities to safely discover and cross reference more details of a candidate's life than some couples learn about one another after years of marriage. These steps will help you identify the reasons to begin or not begin a courtship.

Step 3: Preliminary Fact-Finding
Stepping-Stone Rapport Building

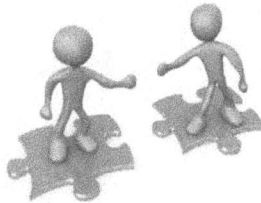

After the candidates and their parents have mutually agreed to discussion guidelines, since the biographies and autobiographies may not have been prepared, the parents can take the opportunity to periodically chat on the phone to share more about their lives. These rapport-building conversations can serve as stepping stones for later collaboration in support of the potential marriage of their adult children--if an engagement and marriage should result. The parents can update their son or daughter with the content of those conversations.

Behind the Curtain

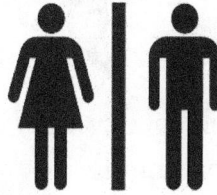

From "behind the curtain" provided by the parents, the candidates can benefit hearing the life stories of their potential parents-in-law. There are several reasons for the candidates and their parents to agree for there to be no direct communication between the candidates until sufficient fact-finding information has been exchanged and discussed between the parties, and until the candidates agree to directly communicate with one another.

One reason is to promote emotional safety. Exploring the possibility of marriage involves hopes and fears and feelings that can be hurt. Therefore, when the candidates remain "behind a curtain," and trusted family members act on their behalf, emotional space and time are provided that can ease the stress of early fact-finding.

Secondly, more honest and meaningful information about the candidates can be vetted prior to any face-to-face meeting. How many stories have you heard about subscribers to online dating and matching websites who were surprised when, after meeting their "match" in person, they discovered their matches' profiles were filled with lies and misrepresentations? Even their physical appearances and profile pictures did not always match.

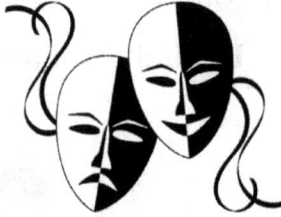

The global research agency *OpinionMatters* surveyed 1000 men and women belonging to various leading dating websites in the US and the UK. The results confirmed what many online daters experience: 53% of the Americans admitted that they had lied on their dating profiles. Also, women lied by 10 percentage points more than men. And Americans lied more than Britons by 9 percentage points. Men lied about their jobs, height, weight, physique and money. Women lied about those factors as well as their age.[111]

A third reason is to assure that any meeting is clearly for the purpose of marriage. It is not to hang out nor to hook up and engage in sexual relations. The willingness to go through *A Better Way To Marry* expresses the seriousness of a potential candidate, another litmus test for marital readiness.

If you are self-matching, a fourth reason for candidates not to directly communicate during this preliminary fact-finding phase is physical and financial safety. Do not become the victim of a "catfish" and suffer financial loss, or emotional or physical harm.

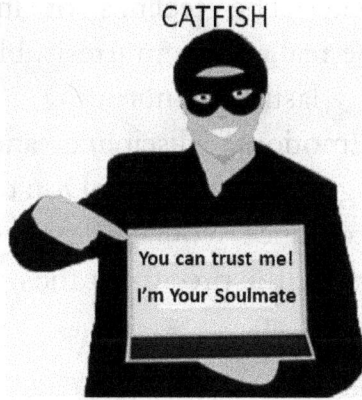

A catfish is a slang term for someone who uses social media like Facebook, Twitter and Instagram to create a false online identity to defraud a victim. Some warning signs that your object of desire may not be who they say they are include: the person you recently met online starts calling you their soulmate, their dating profile photo is beautiful, their Facebook profile has few friends and pictures of people who are not tagged, the person says there has been an accident, cancer, or death in their family, uses bad grammar, and gives repeated excuses why they are unable to have a video chat or meet you personally.[112] Innocent people can fall in love quickly.

Managing Emotions and False Idealization

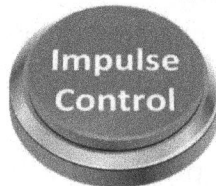

If two singles appear attractive to one another, there is a natural inclination to impulsively start talking to one another with the hope of "connecting" in a very emotional and intimate way. The feelings of intense, passionate attraction may be real and seem irresistible, but they do not translate into lasting, nurturing, reliable marital relationships. Emotional discipline and a process are needed to manage such impulses. Don't make the mistake of trying to convince yourself and others that your euphoric feelings are the proof that the other is "the One."

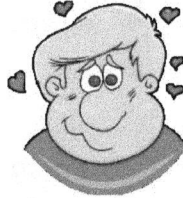

There are likely to be many conflicting emotions to manage. You might feel increasingly hopeful that your efforts would result in an engagement, and, at the same time, fear of making a wrong decision. Even without falling in love, false idealization of a candidate can occur. Idealizing a potential spouse prevents accurately seeing and appreciating the person for who they are and could become and recognizing their traits that need to be complemented. A genuine long-term ideal is for the candidates to become the best that they can become in life--to realize their human potential through marriage. False idealization could mask someone unsuited for marriage.

Once parents exchange their biographies, they can discuss the biography of the other candidate with their son or daughter. Referencing the Three Benchmarks and their Indicators, they can prepare further questions to discuss during the parents' next scheduled phone conversation. After the parents mutually exchange questions and answers, they can huddle again with their son or daughter to discuss the replies. If more questions need to be asked, another discussion can be scheduled. Then each set of parents and their son or daughter can decide whether to continue to the next step.

Step 4: Advanced Fact-Finding

If all the parents and candidates agree to go to the next step, they can exchange the candidates' autobiographies along with other available personality evaluations such as the Flag Page or Myers-Briggs Type Indicator (MBTI) results. With the receipt of added information, it is important for all parties to review it, and to prepare questions that are important to ask when interviewing the candidate.

Preparing for the Interview

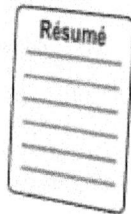

Biographies and autobiographies contain important facts about the candidates and their families that can provide a base line of knowledge from which to prepare important questions for further interviews. While deeply personal in nature, they are likened to resumes that, when combined with interviews, can be used to match applicants with job descriptions in corporations. In fact, businesses use the terms matchmaking, for instance, B2B Matchmaking, www.businessmatchmaking.com, or investor matchmaking. Experienced company hiring managers engaged in job matchmaking know the importance of clear job descriptions and asking good questions.

The Candidate Interview

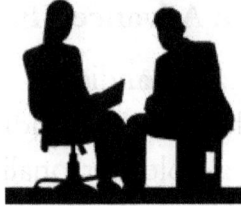

There is a lot of anticipation surrounding the first meeting with the candidate. You can begin with a list of rapport-building questions that promote appreciation and understanding. Asking about the candidate's childhood experiences and current interests can serve as an ice-breaker for discussions.

As more questions are gradually asked, they can become more sensitive in nature. Millennials who expect unlimited access to broad ranges of data should appreciate the importance of disclosure. The goal is to provide the candidates with all information that is reasonably possible so they may make informed marital decisions.

Seeking to put the candidates at ease, you can preface questions with the following: "Marriage is such a serious commitment that thoughtful people discuss important questions that can be sensitive. We would like to ask you some personal questions. If you are offended by any of them, we ask for your patience and forgiveness in advance. You can tell us that you do not want to answer them. Is that okay with you?"

There Can Be Pushback

There are many basic and meaningful questions related to marriage and a candidate's preparedness. *A Better Way To Marry* process can potentially reveal more about a person than one could learn after years of dating or after years of marriage. It is possible, however, that single adults and their parents or advocates, may become defensive and hesitant in revealing their personal lives.

An individual may argue, for example, that since they are not married yet, they don't need to answer your questions, or need not prove themselves ready for marriage. They may be reluctant to divulge personal information, expecting to be trusted without the disclosure, or condition their disclosure upon a promise of commitment for courtship or engagement. Parents and a candidate may be inclined to think that the sooner the two candidates start talking together about marriage, and without asking preliminary "inconvenient" questions, the better. There can be pushback. Therefore, assure that all parties have agreed in advance that consensus—the candidates and their parents (or trusted advisors)—is required to proceed to each next step.

Certainly, the willingness to explore one's life, personality, and goals can be a daunting task. Full disclosure, though, is necessary for single adults to make a well-reasoned and informed decision to marry or not marry. If an individual genuinely desires to develop a marital relationship, they will demonstrate the willingness to do whatever is necessary.

Slower Is Better

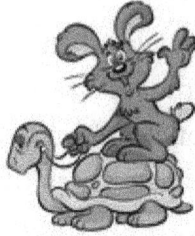

The matchmaking process should not be hurried. Time is needed to navigate through layers of discovery to discern the character and personality of the person being considered as a marriage partner. Proceeding with steady, measured steps can provide insight for how the candidates and their parents make decisions and their capacity to be supportive team players in the extended family. Patience is needed to allow everyone the opportunities to ask the questions they think and feel are important. Impulsive decision making is not a safe, smart, stable basis for choosing a lifelong mate. The rush to say "Yes" could be regretted. Slower is better and can more likely result in a choice that is informed, reliable, and that you can bet your life on.

Keep a Journal

Sufficient time and layers of inquiry are needed to develop a thorough understanding of the candidate being considered. The upfront fact-finding phase of the process can occur over a longer period than anticipated, depending on the families' circumstances.

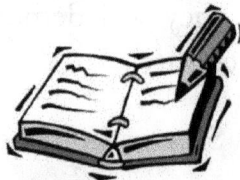

Preparing questions in advance of interviews and maintaining a running journal of conversations help to provide focus during the emotional ups and downs that typically occur in phone and face-to-face discussions. Your notes can also be referenced when writing your assessment of a candidate.

Whether To Meet Just Before the Courtship Decision (Step 5)

Arguments can be made for and against the candidates meeting one-on-one and with their parents before the decision is made to begin a courtship. The unique circumstances will guide that decision.

If the decision is to meet, ask yourselves, "What are the purposes?" Is it to determine whether you feel physical attraction--"chemistry"—the feeling of electricity and butterflies in your stomach? Or is it something else that is prudent? Assure your expectations for a meeting are realistic and not unrealistic. Don't expect a perfect, uncomplicated meeting. Emotions can run high and either of the candidates or their parents might, for example, to everyone's surprise, lose their temper or make awkward or offensive comments that are uncharacteristic of them, which can--in an instant--distort an otherwise accurate and well-documented profile of the other who could become a very good spouse. You or a nervous candidate may talk like a machine gun and not respectfully listen, or may take long, painful pauses before responding to the other.

Regarding attraction: If it is to be lasting in marriage, there must be admiration, the respect and warm approval for what is impressive and worthy in your eyes. What is admirable in your potential spouse deserves your time, effort and patience to discover, recognize and appreciate.

Some young adults (or parents) may presume that they are so discerning that in one or two meetings they can ferret out the basic truth of another, even without the fact-finding steps and selected questions discussed in the previous chapters. Good luck! First impressions and one's feelings are not always correct.

Of course, a candidate's destructive attitudes and behaviors may be very obvious in person, which were not disclosed in their interviews, autobiography, or in their parents' biography. That is reason to acquire reliable third-party opinions of the candidate and their family. Courtship is also a time for verification of what has been discovered thus far.

Some candidates may have already extensively conversed with one another through school, work or other activities. Living in different parts of the country or world, some may never have met or have spoken to one another. If there is considerable distance between the families, decide who would assume the practical burdens such as travel expenses, and impact on one's health. If Skype or other telecommunications are used, remember that visual and auditory distortions can occur during communications.

Step 5: Pre-Courtship
Predicting Future Behavior

When your son or daughter place a very special trust in you to be their mentors and partners to select a lifelong mate, a high level of thoughtfulness, study and dialogue with them are required.

Reasons Not to Start Courtship

After the candidates and their parents have accumulated a considerable amount of useable knowledge about one another, there will come a time to determine whether it is advisable for the two candidates to meet and explore the possibilities of marriage—in other words, courtship! That gets back to the basic question of "what is a healthy human being who is prepared for marriage?" Candidates need not be "perfect" to be healthy and happy together. Marriage, though, is not the place to fix basic character and personality disorders.

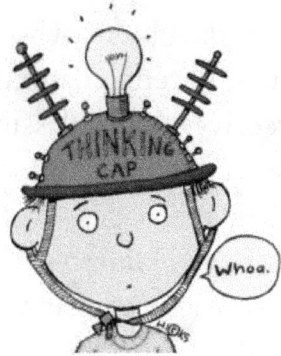

Therefore, some reasons not to recommend two candidates for courtship are:

1) One or both are emotionally and spiritually immature and have not formed a clear identity, or healthy sense of self-worth.

2) Their life goals related to marriage are not defined and/or are frequently changing.

3) They have unrealistic marriage expectations and irreconcilable disagreements.

4) They have no experience being independent.

5) Their desire to marry is to avoid loneliness and leave behind unhappy relationships.

6) One or both may have significant personality or behavior disorders.

Another reason not to recommend courtship is if the desire to marry is just to please others, for instance, parents, friends, or a religious/cultural organization. Sons and daughters, who have a close, healthy relationship with their parents, naturally desire to please their parents and to receive their blessing and approval for marriage. When such parents partner with their children in the formation of their marriages, even when parents genuinely affirm that it is their children's responsibility to make the final decision for whom to marry, it is prudent to double-check the adult child's motivation.

Written Evaluations

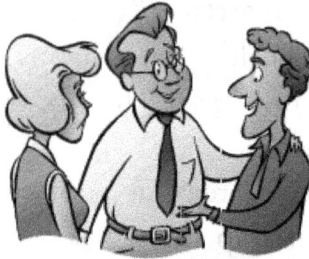

There will come a time after the fact-finding and interviews when the candidates and their parents are ready to evaluate whether to continue into courtship. While the candidates are forming their opinions of one another and their family, they will be curious and may ask, "Dad, Mom... do you think (s)he has or does not have the *potential* to be a loving spouse and reliable life partner for me?" That is also a central question for each candidate to ask themself.

Marriage is a huge, life-changing commitment that requires coherent decisions based on realistic expectations. However authoritative you may think intuition, a revelation, a *spark* or an attraction is to justify a marriage decision, it must still be verified. It is prudent that the candidates and their parents each take the time and effort to prepare a written evaluation.

Draw upon the many sources of information that have been acquired about the candidates and their families: the candidates' biographies and photos prepared by their parents, notes of interviews with the candidates' parents, family members and trusted friends; the candidates' self-reports through their autobiographies, Flag Page summaries and other personality questionnaires, notes from interviews with them, social media (Facebook posts, other), and other helpful information.

The Three Benchmarks and many marriage readiness Indicator questions and answers can provide the framework within which to evaluate the meanings of these sources of information.

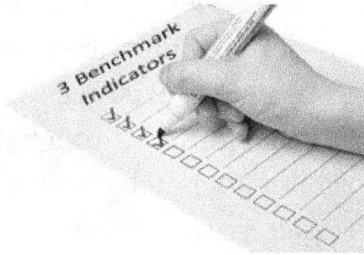

A thoughtfully prepared written assessment can provide an objective evaluation of the strengths, concerns, and threshold challenges that the candidates likely would encounter if they were to marry, and that they could discuss and verify during their personal conversations, if they choose to initiate courtship discussions.

The process of writing a marital evaluation (assessment) may not be easy at first. Remember, though, the questions do not need to be perfectly crafted. The important thing is to identify *patterns* of personality and character behavior, both those that are consistent or inconsistent and contradictory. Accuracy can be improved by triangulating different sources. Many human resource departments in businesses use 360-degree, multi-source-feedback assessments with self-evaluations to improve employee performance.

Is There Potential?

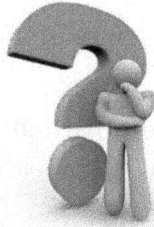

Understanding another human being can be like examining an iceberg, peeling an onion, or bringing an object into camera focus.

Even with the best of interviews and vetting, though, there is no 100 percent guarantee that a marriage will survive the storms and thrive through the years. It is the ultimate responsibility of each couple to live with full integrity to fulfill their marriage vows.

Seeking Consensus

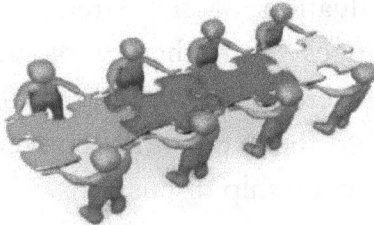

At this stage, it is essential for parents and their son/daughter to review and discuss one another's written assessment of the potential candidate. Discuss whether they agree with their respective evaluations and why or why not. Concurrently, request and discuss the written assessments of the candidate being considered and their parents. Seek consensus as a family whether to begin courtship discussions with the other candidate.

Candidates Decide Whether to Meet

If both candidates and their respective parents agree to proceed to the next step of courtship when the candidates directly communicate, it is important to clarify and confirm what this means for everyone. Ask again, "What are your thoughts about that?" Always check and double check. There may be different interpretations of what the next step means, even if it was initially stated in writing and previously discussed. Send e-mails that seek confirmation of those understandings.

CHAPTER 8

STEP 6:
COURTSHIP TO PRE-ENGAGEMENT

Truth often surfaces in layers, and that can take longer than you think. No one enjoys unpleasant surprises after becoming emotionally involved.

The qualities that really matter in marriage take time to discover, since singles may not even be aware of what they are.

Courtship is the time and process of determining whether to become engaged to marry. If you are single and desiring to marry, during courtship it is important to ask your potential spouse lots of meaningful questions and to verify their answers.

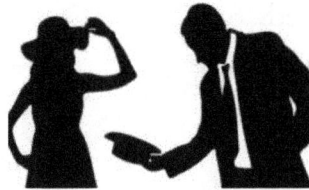

Committing to marriage involves making choices that affect your emotional, spiritual, mental, financial and physical health, your debts, longevity, career, where you live, whether to have children, the merging of two families. Without satisfying answers to basic questions, couples enter blindly into marriage and are very vulnerable.

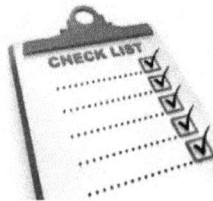

The fact-finding and pre-courtship phase of patiently asking and answering questions, verbally and in writing, can provide marital candidates with in-depth knowledge of one another and a sense of familiarity, before meeting one another in courtship. This chapter explains guidelines that serve as prudent practices during courtship.

Marriage-Connected Dating Begins

Courtship is when "real" dating begins. Its purposes are connected to marriage and for the candidates to

- Verify and confirm whether the previous assessments and assumptions about one another were accurate,
- Directly explore whether they could form a lifelong partnership, and
- Ultimately, determine whether or not to marry.

Disclosure and Verification

A common complaint among singles who use online dating websites is that the listed profiles are often inaccurate or even downright dishonest. During the pre-courtship phase, material facts should be disclosed because they are directly related to the decision to marry. With full, honest disclosure, each candidate can make the personal decision as to whether any disclosed "issues" are manageable or are dealbreakers. If one is committing to a lifelong relationship, one needs to be fully informed as to what that will entail. No one wants unpleasant surprises, especially after becoming emotionally involved.

Don't Rush to Say "Yes" or "No"

While candidates and their parents in the initial steps of *A Better Way To Marry* process are asked to provide accurate disclosures of material facts, courtship is a time to continue their verification. The initial stages are designed to provide safety for all parties and to facilitate honest and meaningful discovery. However, it may occur that a candidate withholds certain facts or relevant details during this phase, deciding to directly disclose them to the candidate during courtship. But that could be problematic and compromising for all parties, especially if the candidate continues to conceal potential dealbreakers.

Let's say that you have been honest and have made full disclosure. What about the person, though, whom you are considering as a potential mate? It is possible that they may be a great performer hiding an addiction, have controlling fantasies, or harbor destructive scripts ready to be activated when in a close intimate relationship.

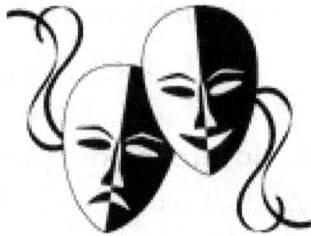

Just as many Internet dating website profiles are filled with lies, what has been written and verbalized in interviews may be very different from what one really believes and practices.

The more sensitive the issues, the more time that is needed for full disclosure and for any concealed problems to be surfaced. Truth often surfaces in layers, and that can take longer than one would think.

Disclosures include whether the candidate has

- Engaged in premarital sex, other sexual activities including pornography, cyber porn, verbal abuse or physical violence against others;
- A sexually transmitted disease (STD) such as gonorrhea, which is common and the CDC has reported may soon be resistant to all antibiotics and be untreatable;[113]
- Committed a crime (misdemeanor or felony);
- Has or had addictions or compulsive behaviors, or mental or physical health diagnoses or issues, for instance, depression, suicidal thoughts, anxiety.

Can you imagine how much more difficult it would be for a man and woman to directly ask those questions and verify their answers during (false) romantic love-based dating when the excitement and passion of physical attraction override normal rational thinking, and when fun and pleasure are the priorities of dating?

False Chemistry vs. True Chemistry

Some of you may be thinking, "Where is the chemistry, the *passion* -- the feeeellling in this process of courtship!?" Well, the chemistry of attraction does bud and evolve as respect, admiration and trust grow.

Yet, at the same time, are initial feelings of attraction a reliable basis for making decisions that have lifelong consequences? Romantic feelings can be very wrong.

Psychologist John Van Epp references studies of nearly 10,000 married couples from 33 countries who assert that mutual attraction and love feelings are prerequisites for choosing a partner and for marriage to become successful.

He warns that chemistry is "not a good judge of character," that it "sees what it wants to see," and "is not constant even in the best of relationships."[114]

Women disappointed with the dating scene confide that they had grown up believing that a "divine spark" must be experienced as a precondition to marry. Writer Lori Gottlieb regrets that she and her friends "walked away from uninspiring relationships that might have made us happy in the context of a family."[115]

Generally, it is recognized that males are visually-oriented and often overestimate physical appearance over other qualities. Have you ever wondered why some individuals are attracted to "bad boys" or "crazy girls" who are exciting and adventurous but also dangerous and destructive?

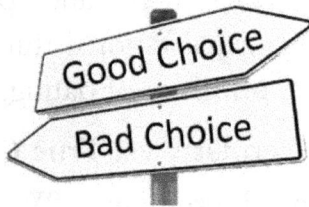

First impressions can be misleading. Much of Jane Austen's novel *Pride and Prejudice* is about Elizabeth Bennet's first and wrong impressions of Mr. Darcy, due to her overconfidence and false pride in her own perceptions.

It is worth reemphasizing the fact that marriages based on (false) romantic love teeter on a platform of unrealistic expectations and fantasies. The intense feelings of excitement and romantic attraction are given undue priority and often are the overriding factor in human relationships. Beyond looks, other factors such as charisma, wealth and status may weigh disproportionately in the development of early relationships.

Consider the nature of "chemistry." There is false chemistry and true chemistry. False chemistry is the untenable and temporary roller coaster of emotions experienced in (false) romantic love, from a racing heart rate of excitement and longing which escalates, implodes and then disappears, leaving a disappointing aftertaste of regret, loss and possibly depression, the falling-out-of-love experience. The experiences are real but are not nurturing and cannot sustain a marriage.

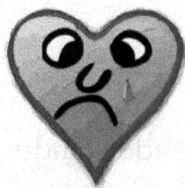

True chemistry, on the other hand, is sustainable and nurturing. It must be developed, though, over time. *A Better Way To Marry* process can stimulate natural attraction and admiration. Making the efforts to reveal who they are through their writings, interviews and other activities, candidates can demonstrate that they are serious and have endearing and admirable qualities. Trust develops and enables a potential mate to take the risk of being honest and emotionally close. Trust and admiration stimulate attraction, fondness and affection, especially when both your strengths and weaknesses are accepted. That is a more solid basis for passion and true chemistry to be sustained and grow in a marriage.

The chemistry of attraction is an important component of marital relationships and can serve to further connect and support the intimacy of a couple. However, it must be approached with caution and the appropriate kindling must be placed to assure a sustainable fire.

If you are single, whether you collaborate with your parents and family who serve as trusted advisors, or decide to self-match, there are useful and safe practices to consider when dating a prospective mate.

Take Measured Steps to Build Trust

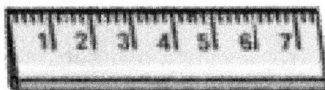

Making an informed choice to marry means that you understand to whom and to what you are committing. The qualities that really matter in marriage take time to discover since singles may not even be aware of what they are. A foundation of trust must be built so a single adult can safely step forward toward commitment. A marriage candidate must earn trust. When a candidate writes an honest and well-prepared autobiography and an honest, well-balanced profile, they fortify and expand that foundation of trust. Trust is developed through meaningful conversations when the candidates take the risk of revealing their true selves, their hopes and dreams, likes and dislikes, wants and needs, strengths and weaknesses, fears, successes and disappointments, as well as their readiness for marriage.

Just as honesty is important for establishing trust, active and respectful listening is required to understand the meaning of what the other reveals. It takes time to develop genuine and effective communication.

Learning to Dance

Singles exploring a potential marriage are best reminded that individuals have different emotional and intellectual speeds, and different expectations. Learning whether you can live together is like learning to dance with a partner.

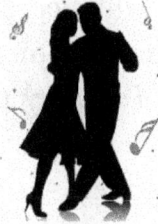

Your individual sense of rhythm in conversation can be different and these rhythms can even change over time.

Be careful not to judge a person by first impressions: "His first question was, 'Mac or PC?' He was Mac and I am PC. I don't like Macs." "Her handshake was too aggressive!" "She is nerdy and awkward!"

Don't Judge by First Impressions

He may accidentally step on your toes (and you on his toes) instead of sweep you off your feet, or unintentionally make a remark that is hurtful. In the early stages of meeting a candidate who might become your spouse, they may be nervous, have an adrenaline rush and talk like a machine gun without pause: "He just talked nonstop about himself and his new computer game. He did not ask questions about me." On the other hand, nervousness may trigger long stretches of silence which can be uncomfortable. Give the nervousness time to subside and for the pace of talking to normalize. Whether the pace of the conversational dance becomes too fast or too slow, be patient with the person who has invested much to get to this point in courtship.

Too much or too little talking does not mean the person would not be a wonderful life partner. Allow time for your candidate to express themself, and time for both of you to reflect and determine whether you can synchronize your lives together. One happily married man who has gone through *A Better Way To Marry* process concurs, "During courtship, she was very nice; but I was awkward. Fortunately, she was patient and discovered that I am a good person. Since then, she says that I have become a good husband for her." Also, be patient with yourself. After all, no person is fully formed when beginning a marriage. Managing differences and expectations toward meaningful goals is a skill.

Whether you believe that marriage is the most important life decision or only one among many, it does have long-term consequences and impacts your emotional life, financial life, family life, and physical health. Make a fully informed decision.

Do Not Let Physical Passions Betray You

At the beginning of courtship, it is important to have a predetermined agreement for physical boundaries, i.e., no sex before marriage. Two candidates may immediately hit it off and experience strong and overwhelming feelings of physical attraction.

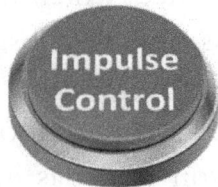

Those impulses must be managed, however, because it can be very damaging to the decision-making process and the relationship if physical boundaries are prematurely crossed. The blindness of passionate love can mask underlying problems that, if left undetected, can destroy a relationship and your marriage. If unrestrained freedom and immediate pleasure are prioritized over the long-term consequences of premature sexual relationships, enduring emotional pain and scars, and loss of trust and marriage can result.

Ask All the Important Questions: Expectations

During courtship, it is foolish to think that you should not ask personal questions before an engagement or a lifelong commitment like marriage. Yet, it is common for couples contemplating marriage to skip over necessary questions. For a variety of reasons, one or both may think, "I could not ask those questions or talk about that! We are not even engaged; it would be presumptuous of me to talk about where we might live, who would move to the other's city, how each of us could pursue our educations and careers. Also, if I am not clear about what I want to do in my life, how can I even ask those questions?" Candidates may not want to appear presumptuous or scare away a potential candidate by asking very direct and personal questions.

Understanding another's expectations, strengths and weaknesses, hopes and fears does not happen just by spending time together.

Asking essential and difficult questions and observing how a potential mate responds and collaborates with you to seek your common well-being are absolutely important. It is much easier to probe into central marriage questions by first asking them from behind the curtain of safety during the preliminary fact-finding discussions.

Sticking points are common; however, the depth of knowing yourself and a potential mate can deepen if you skillfully collaborate to identify the road ahead, "If we were to marry, how would we live?"

Synchronizing Two Lives?

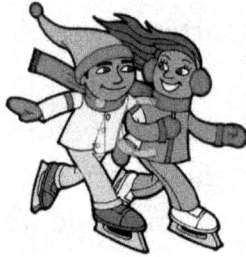

As candidates sense increasing possibilities for a "match" and engagement, they best keep their feet on the ground and review the practical realities of the road ahead. They can forecast the future by brainstorming how they would pursue their careers or continued education, where they might live, and by drafting a general outline of different shared lifestyles together during the next three to five years.

If there are important long-term decisions that you have not resolved, such as your career focus, you have an opportunity for the person you are considering to marry to demonstrate how willing and able they would be as your helpmate. They can reveal whether they are willing and able to go from "me" to "we."

There will be many times in your life when your next steps are not clear and are full of uncertainties and dilemmas. You and your future partner will need to find your way together. The process of managing life's dilemmas is often as important as the decisions made to resolve those dilemmas.

Imagining a Life Together

Imagining and forecasting the future with a potential mate is like building a home. We desire that it be safe and sound. Home builders and contractors are often fearful of city inspectors scrutinizing their work, fearful that they would be told that their efforts do not comply with public health and safety standards and that corrections must be made. Similarly, young, romantically involved couples don't want to be told that they are incorrectly structuring their personal lives.

We desire homes that are safe, healthy and comfortable places to live. We rely upon solid foundations and wall connections that comply with minimum building and safety regulations to withstand storms and earthquakes. We expect that our homes' support systems such as heating and air conditioning, plumbing and electrical will provide warmth in winters, maintain coolness during hot summers, and not transmit toxic elements into the air or water through the plumbing.

Failed marriages are like inadequately built homes. They were blown off their foundations when adverse winds buffeted their relationship. Marriages can become unlivable when a couple stops or fails to invest in the foundation of their relationship. While a marriage should be filled with empathy, forgiveness, admiration, affection and trust, space

179

and support for personal growth, failed marriages often harbor emotional environments that are cold, toxic, and overwhelmed by stress.

Check the Foundation

Before committing to an engagement and marriage, do your best to assure that if you were to marry the candidate, your marriage would be structurally sound and have adequate support systems. When homebuyers view Open Houses for sale, few consider looking at the foundations of those homes.

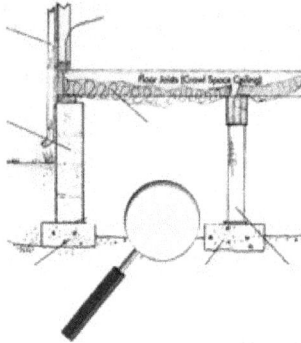

They are preoccupied with how beautiful the rooms look and the available upgrades. Foundations are not easy to see, nor are they usually easy and desirable places to access. Too often, individuals are inclined to make their marriage assessments based on appearances and first impressions, without conducting adequate inspections.

The intense feelings of excitement and passion are given undue priority. When in love, the mystical force of "love" will solve all things...so one thinks. The largest and most important investments in life--marriage and the purchase of a home--are often based primarily on unmanaged impulses and presumptions that are not realistic or well-informed.

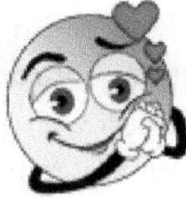

For various reasons, there may be reluctance to talk about the future: it could be a wild-eyed sense that asking questions would diminish the romantic adventure or the delusion that everything will be perfect, that "love will solve everything." More often, though, it may be a fear of what may be discovered that would threaten getting married or threaten one's dreams.

Careers and Where to Live

It is likely that both a husband and wife would pursue a career. There is a price to pay for each career choice and place to live. Unless both live in the same area, one of them would need to eventually move to the other spouse's city. That could mean a big risk for the one who moves, especially if job opportunities are few in their career field. It could mean separating from all that is familiar and supportive, and possibly moving away from a much more pleasant environment. A sense of loss and heartfelt pain could be experienced. Assure that the advantages and disadvantages of each decision are understood, appreciated and mutually agreed upon.

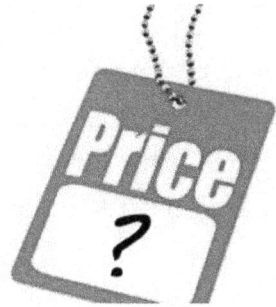

Couples should discuss:

- Where would we both live so each of us could pursue our career or continue our education?
- How could we connect with one another's family, friends and supportive community?
- If one of us has a demanding work or school schedule and periods of limited personal time, how could we assure that we both have sufficient emotional support, that we maintain regular communication, and that we do not turn away from each other?
- How would the highest and best physical, emotional and spiritual health of each of us be furthered?

Individual career and living location choices come with a price that is paid as a couple and by their children, not just one person. What is that price? It is not only financial, but also time spent apart and loneliness. What price would the husband ask his wife to pay for him to pursue his career? What price would the wife ask her husband to pay for her to pursue her career?

Discussing Money

Money can be a divisive factor. It can represent something different to each partner in a marriage. One partner may view money as security, a means to eliminate worry and stress. The other spouse could regard money as freedom and pleasure.

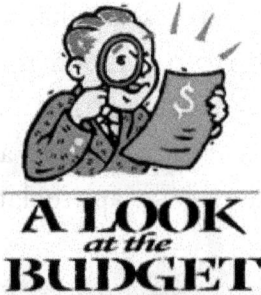
A LOOK *at the* **BUDGET**

Huge student loans are common today. If one or both candidates have a $25,000 to $100,000 student

182

loan debt, what would be the monthly repayment? Could they manage it—financially and emotionally?

Spreadsheet Forecasting

The candidates in courtship could forecast how life would be together by drafting different budgets for different lifestyles in the different cities where they are most likely to live. Estimate all living expenses and debt repayments. If you work within a big city, is it better to rent within the city where rents are higher, or commute to more affordable areas?

Spreadsheet forecasting can channel you to confront the premises of your dreams, and your concepts of success and happiness. Define the bases of your American Dream.

Surface your expectations. Is your bottom line expectation that you must "have it all" (fulfilling career, marriage, family, travel, sports, etc.) and "at the same time?" Do you regard anything less than that as "settling for less?" Manage your debt. Do not let it manage you.

Parents and In-Laws

A healthy, on-going relationship with your parents and in-laws is important. Candidates can ask themselves, "What obligations would we have to our families?" Consider, for instance, the obligations of children to respect and care for elderly parents, to fulfill extended family traditions, and "honor-shame codes," which are part of the societal fabric in most of the world, not just Arab and Asian cultures. Parents from those cultures may consciously or unconsciously presume that their children living in a Western society would conform to their view of filial piety. For example, Asian parents may expect their newly married children and their spouses to financially provide for them, which could be a very disruptive surprise for a non-Asian fiancé.

We learned about Ralph, born and raised in the US, who was dating Josephina, a lovely lady who immigrated from the Philippines. Her father and mother, in their late 50s, were financially supported by their other children living in the Philippines. When Ralph and Josephina were planning for their marriage, Josephina's sister and other siblings decided that her wedding should be held in Hawaii and that Ralph should pay for it, as well as pay for the travel expenses for all of Josephina's family living in the Philippines to attend the wedding. Ralph also learned that after the marriage, he would be expected to contribute "his share" toward Josephina's parents' lifestyle. Can you imagine how Ralph reacted when he discovered that?

Family-care questions are difficult to ask and answer. Consider:

- Would care for elderly or sick parents fall on the shoulders of you or your prospective spouse? Would you accept that?
- How do you feel about assuming financial or other responsibility for your future parents-in-law?

It is important that those expectations be known, disclosed, discussed, and mutually agreed upon, if a marriage is to be formed. While the marriage of two persons is commonly recognized as the marriage of two families, expectations for one's future role in another family may differ.

Special Needs Siblings

Whether or not one believes that the marriage of a couple is the marriage of two families, inevitably, siblings do affect a marriage. Concern and involvement, whether in small or big ways, in the care of special needs siblings is part of the marriage commitment. Any couple contemplating marriage should include what that care and involvement could mean in their potential engagement discussions and not leave it unspoken. Special needs children are the concern for all members of the family. Consider asking:

- Do you have any siblings with physical or mental disabilities who would need assistance from family in the future?

- How do you envision your relationship with that sibling changing over time, and do you anticipate assuming a caregiver role for that sibling?

Children

Discuss whether you can agree on whether to have children, when and how many.

Identify Dilemmas and Your Non-Negotiables

With the goal of supporting one another's highest and best well-being, the previous sections highlighted dilemmas and common conflicts encountered in marriages: family, vocation, money/debts, in-laws, and children.

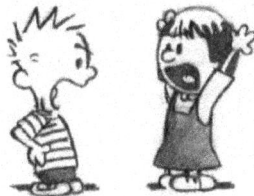

Every couple carries into marriage a set of issues and conflicts that are common to others and unique to them. The important thing is to skillfully and compassionately manage those issues. Burying one's head in the sand or denying those issues can aggravate them. A couple needs to know in advance how they would handle such dilemmas and conflicts if they are to make informed decisions to marry. It is prudent for each individual to review and ask themself:

- What are my dealbreakers?" "Have they changed?
- What must a prospective mate agree with to live with me?
- Are these reasonable expectations?

Agree How to Manage Conflict

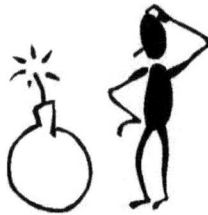

All marriages encounter conflicts and dilemmas that need to be managed, usually within the context of busy schedules, limited finances and many uncertainties. At some point during courtship discussions, to prevent unpleasant surprises, and before any commitment to an engagement occurs, it is prudent for a couple to agree on how they would address their basic conflicts and dilemmas. The more you can discover and agree in advance on the best ways to build a marriage and a home, the greater will be your potential for marital satisfaction.

Third Alternative Solutions

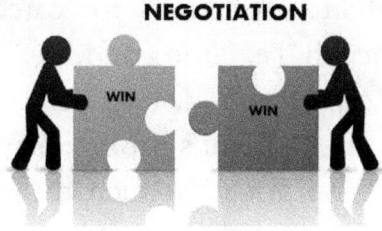

NEGOTIATION

Covey's "third alternative" to solve professional and personal difficulties is a method that can help you do that. It is an essential process and skill that can result in win-win outcomes for couples. Adaptations of this method have been used in business, government and nonprofit sectors with a high degree of success.[116]

The basic idea is that two singles often approach marriage with different perspectives about how to address career, intimacy, money, family, in-laws, faith, lifestyle, children, and other daily concerns. It is possible to discover through a creative, systematic process a new and better solution that includes the best ideas and benefits for both candidates.

The "Double T" Diagram

Draw a "T" diagram with an additional column. One candidate's name heads one column and the other's name heads the other column. The third column is titled "Win-Win", the third alternative solution.

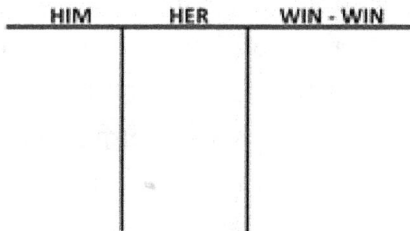

HIM	HER	WIN - WIN

One candidate, the "Speaker," begins by explaining their "big picture" of life aspirations for career, family, public service, travel, health, i.e., "the good life." Then the other--the "Listener/Responder"—listens with empathy and then verbally repeats the Speaker's aspirations until the Speaker is able to say, "You got it!" which means that they have been sufficiently heard and understood. Such exercises in communication are likened to "active listening," "empathic listening," and used in the "Indian talking stick" process.

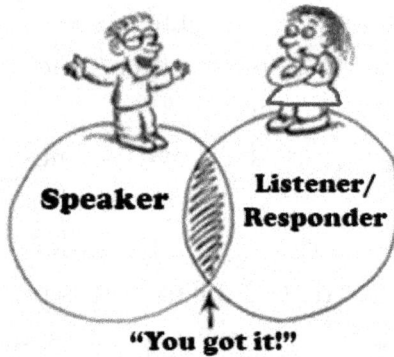

"You got it!"

When the Speaker's aspirations have been satisfactorily verbalized, record them in the corresponding column and then reverse the roles until both participants feel that their aspirations have been recorded to their satisfaction.

Next "brainstorm" win-win options that would achieve both candidates' aspirations. Write all of your ideas on separate pieces of paper during this phase, even if an option initially seems crazy and out of the ballpark. At this stage do not offer your opinions of the pros or cons, advantages or disadvantages of each option.

Since all of an individual's aspirations cannot always be realized at the same time, and it would be especially difficult for both marriage partners to realize all their aspirations at the same time, dilemmas will become apparent. That would lead to discussions involving "Who would support the other, how, when and why?"

After brainstorming all the options, discuss the pros and cons of each option. Choose the best option(s) that is a win-win for both of you, which is the third alternative solution. Write them in the Win-Win column. This process can help a couple to synchronize their lives. It is an important skill in marriage and requires self-discipline, patience, humility, empathy, and the capacity to move from "me" to "we."

Some conflicts and dilemmas in marriage are easier to manage than others. Alternatively, prospective marriage partners may feel disrespected, unappreciated, and experience resentment, if they do not allow themselves the opportunity to participate in a genuine collaborative process.

Can You Be Complementary?

In addition to assessing whether you could collaborate on a general life course together, it is important to consider how your strengths and weaknesses may complement one another.

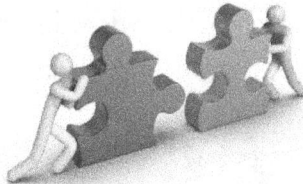

One of the roles of a spouse is to be a helpmate, to complement a weakness or an imbalance with the other's strength. You must know what to help, though, if you are to knowingly commit to it.

Candidates are advised to honestly identify their imperfections. Indeed, it is difficult for humans to do that and to manage them. Common imperfections are tendencies to be impatient, overcritical, disorganized or overcommitted, or impulsive when it comes to an unhealthy eating lifestyle. Consider asking:

- Are you aware of your imperfections and those of the other person you are considering as your potential spouse?
- What would your potential spouse be committing to help you with, for example, are you overly self-critical?
- Do you adequately recognize your differences and how you could complement one another? Are these differences acceptable?

Marry for the Right Reasons

Marry for the right reasons, not the wrong reasons. Sounds like common sense, doesn't it? Many people, though, marry knowing from the beginning that something is wrong and they should not marry their fiancé/fiancée, but do it anyway. Some marry out of fear that there are no other "good ones" available, or that they might lose out on a possible good match if they decided not to marry.

Marriage, however, should ideally not be approached

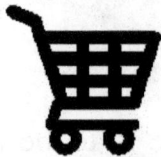

like shopping, thinking, "If it looks like a good buy, get it. Try it when you get home. If it doesn't fit, return it to the store and get your money back." This is the beta marriage attitude.

Reason Neutralized by Passion and Fantasies

Perhaps you do not need to be reminded, but the logic of marrying for the right reasons can easily be neutralized by the rush of illusory chemistry and dysfunctional (fatal) attraction. Many people appreciate this in theory but fall for it anyway.

At some point during this pre-engagement stage, more information may not reveal more meaningful insight because bubbling beneath the surface of conscious awareness you may be comparing the other candidate with your unconscious checklist of features for your ideal mate, your "type", which might be Mr. or Ms. Fantasy.

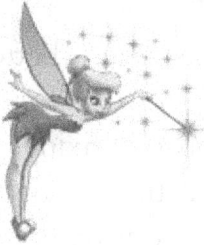

Hopefully, those presumptions would have been surfaced and honestly resolved during the previous stages. Do not underestimate the power of those assumptions and fantasies to override common sense and good judgment. The person you are considering as a mate may be comparing you, too, with such unrealistic ideals.

Be careful, therefore, about rejecting someone who may not fit perfectly into your "type." Reflect on the underlying purposes behind your expectations in a spouse. Expectations of sustained, high levels of euphoric passion in marriage will not result in happiness.

On the other hand, it is important to listen to your intuition and heed warning signs during courtship. Don't be blind.

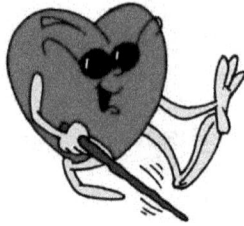

Look out for indications of insincerity, addiction, or a controlling or jealous personality. Just as many Internet dating website profiles are filled with lies, what has been written and verbalized in interviews may be very different from what one really believes and practices.

To Become a Better Person

Marrying someone who can help you become a better person, should be distinguished from the idea of marrying for you "to be fixed" or with the intention of "fixing" a potential spouse. Parents can explain in their written assessments of candidates who are being considered as potential spouses for their adult children why they appear to be complementary. For instance, the tendency to be over exuberant could be tempered and balanced by the steadiness of the other; seriousness could be complemented by the lighted-heartedness of the other; the stiff, logical, rational tendencies of one could be complemented by the artistic sensibilities of the other.

Sounding Board

Parents may have conflicting ideas about their involvement or the involvement of the other parents during this courtship and pre-engagement stage. They may be thinking, "We have given our opinion and green light. Our daughter is smart enough and can figure things out without any more help from us; we won't say a thing or

192

even ask, 'How are things progressing?'" Those parents may presume that the other parents should do the same and say nothing.

It is certainly possible that parents may unwittingly, and with good intentions, be disruptive. Parents may be very confident that a candidate is a great match and push prematurely for a decision. However, they are not marrying the candidate. Positive comments may add to the pressure their son or daughter experiences while evaluating a potential mate. An overzealous father or mother can cause a son or daughter to feel conflicted between pleasing their parents and making a decision for themselves.

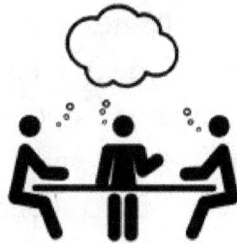

At the same time, parents can be a helpful sounding board during the courtship process, listening to their adult son's/daughter's perceptions of the prospective mate and providing, as needed, good questions to consider. Having parents as trusted advisors and partners who serve as a sounding board can help you sort through your feelings and expectations, doubts, and your experiences with the potential mate. This is one of the roles of elders in families- -to support their members to successfully transition from various stages in life, including marriage. As the positives begin to mount, and natural attraction moves one toward a "yes," it is important that your passion not short circuit due diligence and good sense.

Parents can also help their children clarify and manage their understandings of happiness, success, aspirations and dreams central to life, which are connected to their sense of self, purpose and meanings. *These perceptions often change over time.* Your ideal career and your ideal mate at age 16 may be different at 18, 21, 27 and beyond. Just as one's "type"—i.e., ideal mate--might have been based on unrealistic expectations, one's concepts of success with a life partner may also be unrealistic and instead be a path to loneliness.

Before Saying "Yes" To an Engagement

If and when the candidates are inclined to give a green light to proceed to the next step, which would be an engagement, as a matter of due diligence, it would be prudent for them and jointly with their parents to review their engagement decision to confirm that it was fully informed and based on realistic expectations of one another in marriage. This is similar to the pre-marriage counseling required by some churches and synagogues for couples planning to marry. It is different in that it would occur before a decision to be engaged to marry.

An Inter-Family Discussion

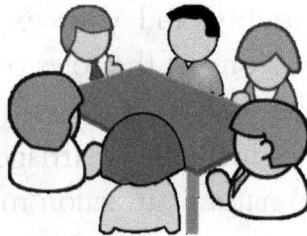

Additionally, it could be done not from the standpoint of a counseling relationship, but rather within the context of a continued commitment to mentorship and the process of learning together.

Parents can request that each of them propose basic questions for a family discussion. The idea is that the prospective fiancé and fiancée and their parents would answer the same questions. Anyone could decline to answer any question. It is an opportunity for group learning, which ideally would continue after a wedding and throughout the many stages of marriage and family life.

Assure Everyone Is on Board

Assure from the beginning, though, that as part of creating exploratory discussion guidelines in Step 2, that everyone is on board with this step and understands its benefits. Otherwise, there might be push back, for instance, the person proposing the "family discussion" might be accused of controlling the process.

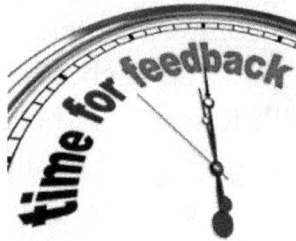

Even when the family discussion is agreed upon in advance in Step 2, either the parents or a candidate may resent answering questions that may be difficult for them to answer. They may be emotionally fixed on going straight to the altar without completing due diligence. Thus, when more questions are asked, they may regard them as a nuisance or a threat. Parents, too, may not want to be involved in the discussions because the questions may be difficult and challenging for them.

Therefore, be diplomatic and patient. It is a good idea to regularly ask, "What are your thoughts?" Safe and meaningful progress depends upon all parties recognizing the value of honest discussion about the basics of marriage. Slower is better. Take whatever time is needed to decide.

Pre-Engagement Family Discussions

Realize, too, that parents can share nuggets of wisdom that benefit everyone. Marriage researchers like John Gottman confirm that nuggets of wisdom about love and marriage dwell within everyday married folks. [117] The research findings of three professors of psychiatry, M.D.s Thomas Lewis, Fari Amini, and Richard Lannon conclude that there is no science of love in their profession of psychiatry, and while academic discoveries in other disciplines such as neurodevelopment, evolutionary theory, psychopharmacology, neonatology, experimental psychology, and computer sciences are important, "[h]uman lives form the richest repository of …the mysteries of love."[118] Researchers have recognized that the stories of ordinary and emotionally intelligent couples contain wisdom that can apply broadly to other marriages.

Here are some questions that could be among those to discuss as part of inter-family discussions:

- Do you know what you do not know about marriage?
- Why are marriages in trouble and why do they fail? Why would your prospective marriage not fail? What are reasons your marriage (the parents) have succeeded?

- What are 12 reasons why you want to marry (the other candidate)? Parents explain the 12 reasons they desire to continue their marriage.
- Why do men and women commit domestic violence?
- Do you have a personal emotional, spiritual, physical safety net that can be used in your future marriage?
- Politics and religion can divide or unite. Do your views differ from one another? Why so? Is it that one of you has more values or principles than the other; or are certain views not regarded as right or principled? Are they reconcilable? How so?
- What are the strengths and weaknesses of one another (candidate to candidate, husband to wife [parents])?
- Have you clarified the unrealistic expectations of one another that could lead to unhappiness in your prospective marriage? Parents answer whether they have or had unrealistic expectations of one another.
- Why do men and women commit adultery?
- Do you complement one another? How so? How could you be a helpmate to one another?
- Do you share the same standards regarding a healthy lifestyle, for instance, diet, exercise, alcohol, sleep, etc.? If not, how could they be reconciled?
- Is "being in-love" the measure of true love in marriage? If so, why? If not, why so? What is true love in the context of marriage?
- Why is there a fascination with romance? What is true romance? In what forms would you like to experience romance?

- How would you describe the road ahead in marriage and family life — the adjustments that each of you will be asked to make, for example, from being a husband to a father, wife to a mother; blending family, work, public service?
- What are the marital skills that each of you have or do not have? Are you prepared to maintain and develop them; for example, take classes to develop conflict management skills?
- What are the hopes and dreams of one another and how will you support one another to fulfill those dreams?
- What are the skills necessary to be a contributing member of an extended family?
- Do you have recurring disagreements with one another? If so, how might you manage them?

Benefits of Pre-Engagement Family Discussions

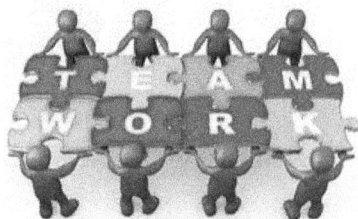

This type of family discussion can be a positive, learning, and nurturing experience. Asking and honestly answering basic questions has real benefits: it can build trust and understanding needed for future collaboration after a wedding. It is a capacity-building exercise for patience, empathy and trust. It can also raise warning signs that, if not responsibly addressed, could be regretted after a decision to marry.

You can utilize any form of communication that best serves the two families for group discussions. For families unable to meet together at a common table due to living considerable distances apart, illness or other reasons, you could conduct discussions over the telephone or through online video streaming applications such as Skype and Google Hangout.

While technology can be helpful, if not well managed, it could also create some unintended misperceptions. Consider how you may come across to others when communicating through a computer webcam. Moving forward to the computer webcam to better hear the discussion may cause your face to become distorted, and combined with bright lighting, may result in your face appearing like an interrogator. Occasionally resting your chin on your fist could give the impression of being disinterested. Be mindful of the images and impressions that you create on the computer screen and make adjustments as needed.

CHAPTER 9

STEP 7:
ENGAGEMENT AND
PRE-MARRIAGE PREPARATION

Fire, ready, aim?

The beginning of an engagement is ideally when a couple memorialize their well-reasoned commitments to live their lives together "in sickness and in health." This chapter proposes practical considerations, activities and preparations before the wedding that may surprise you. It continues the measured, trust building process of Step 6.

Don't Fire, Ready, Aim

Once the decision to become engaged is made, it is commonly thought that the two single adults have *crossed the finish line*, and that it is time for them to spread the good news on Facebook and Twitter, surf wedding websites, fan through bridal magazines, buy a wedding dress and a tuxedo, and plan the wedding. The reality, though, is that there are still some important things to do.

Western engagements often follow a *fire, ready, aim* series of events: a couple is considered officially engaged as fiancée and fiancé *when* the "big question is popped" and the woman accepts the engagement ring as it is slipped onto her finger.

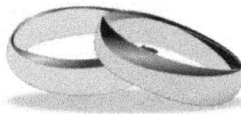

The circular ring symbolizes eternity with the promise of commitment, fidelity and true love.

Yet, it is commonly thought that *then* a couple begins to plan their life together and informs their families of their decision. That is *fire, ready, aim.* If couples are to make fully informed commitments, how can they do that without fully understanding to what they are committing?

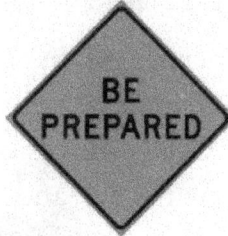

If the symbolism of the ring is to be taken seriously and internalized, then meaningful reflection, discussion and agreements are needed *before* commitments are made. It should be *ready, aim, fire.* Therefore, make sure that you are ready to be formally engaged before rushing to tell others that you are engaged. Marriages often fail before they begin because couples rush forward with unrealistic expectations.

Engagement Not a Trial Period

The engagement period before the wedding is not a trial period to determine whether the couple really wants to get married to one another and can commit to a life together. An engagement is the beginning of two individuals and their two families committing and linking their lives in truly profound ways. Create an engagement commitment ceremony to initiate and formalize the commitments to one another.

Linking Two Families

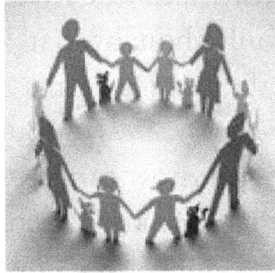

From a multi-generational perspective, today broader family commitments and skills are needed. The consequences of the Great Recession, such as a long-term increase in employment and income inequality, demographic changes, and strains on the Social Security Fund and health care systems necessitate meaningful family collaborations to develop mutual support. [119] The Pew Research Center reports that Millennials are the "first in the modern era to have higher levels of student loan debt, poverty and unemployment, and lower levels of wealth and income" than the two previous generations at the same stage of life. [120] Those seismic economic and social shifts have brought into question the exaggerated expectations of the American Dream, that the lifestyle of each next generation will be better than their parents'. Buying a modest home and maintaining a healthy lifestyle and family connections are more difficult than they were in the past.

It is important to approach marriage not with naïve idealism but realistic optimism and a prudent approach to extended family development where to err is human and to forgive is divine. If couples are adequately prepared for marriage, they can enjoy realistic optimism for fulfilling and meaningful futures. Their parents can also share such realistic optimism for their children. At the same time, parents desire to leave a meaningful legacy of family unity.

The Classic Challenge

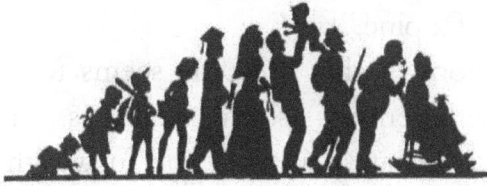

That being said, today parental optimism is countered by popular pessimistic presumptions that generational gaps and divisive conflicts are normal. Strong links in the chain of families are not regarded as the norm. Few families extend beyond three generations in terms of preserving material and spiritual wealth.

The classic challenge of each generation is for the

- Elder generation to transfer wealth--the best of culture, values, ethics, faith, philosophy, as well as real and personal property--to the next generation, and for

- The next generation to receive, preserve and pass it on to the next generation.

One need not be a family scholar to realize that it is difficult for in-laws and extended families to cooperate, not just between three generations, but also within single generations.

Wisdom Recognized

It is easier to expect next generation advancements in technology than in people. It is not common today to consider the possibility of positively influencing seven generations of families. It was, though, a principle of Iroquois Indian elders that guided their decision-making: "In every deliberation, we must consider the impact on the seventh generation…even if it requires having skin as thick as the bark of a pine."[121]

The wisdom of this principle seems to be mirrored in the twentieth-century social sciences, in law firms specializing in estate planning, and in wealth management consulting services, which learned that a shared vision, virtues and values, healthy family relationships, elders, and traditions were required for families and a society to perpetuate themselves at the most fundamental level.

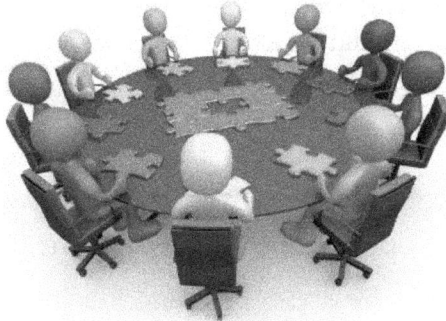

Each new generation must buy into those ideas. Hughes's research and experiences in consulting for multi-generational family businesses provide examples of how it can be done.[122]

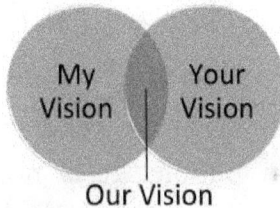

Engagement Commitment Ceremony

An activity that can strengthen the intention for enduring intergenerational cooperation and development is an engagement commitment ceremony. Organize this ritual to clarify and memorialize a couple's and their families' shared commitments. As pre-engagement mentoring discussions can be helpful to strengthen a couple's preparation for marriage, so can a well-prepared engagement ceremony.

Within the ceremony, a couple and their parents join together to stretch their collective imaginations to create a shared vision that extends far beyond into the future—seven generations, longer than any of them will live.

Most of us can visualize the peaceful unity of three generations, as in a Normal Rockwell painting of happy children, their parents and grandparents patiently sitting around a Thanksgiving table watching the carving of the ceremonial golden-brown turkey.

Now from there, envision great grandchildren. It is a little more difficult, isn't it? So, seven generations--150 years or more--is quite a leap in thought and imagination. Such long-term thinking is necessary, though, for those who plant trees in state parks, design planned residential communities, and regional infrastructure developments such as bridges and highways. Protection and preservation of the waters, the air and the earth also require long-term planning. If such intention is required for environment design and infrastructure, why not apply this level of foresight for our families?

Family Covenants

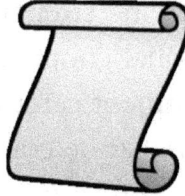

When a man and woman form a marriage, they establish kinship between themselves and between their two families. Their engagement ceremony is an opportunity for their two families to intentionally begin their kinship relationship as partners and with a thoughtfully considered vision that is clear, meaningful to them, and shared. Jointly planning the engagement ceremony can provide a framework that furthers that purpose.

The following are possible core components for an engagement ceremony:

- Reading the engagement ceremony's purpose, and
- Family Covenants, which are a combination of the (a) Engaged Couple's Covenants, (b) the Parents' Covenants, and (c) a Joint Inter-Family Covenant.

They are essentially vision and mission statements. The agenda can include testimonies, music, symbolic rituals such as the exchange of rings and gifts, inspirational readings, humor and group photos.

Building Links Between Families

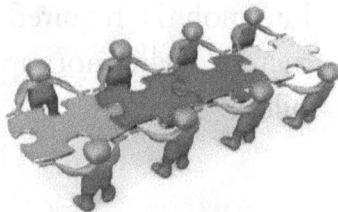

The Covenants are reciprocal pledges of commitments that continue the process of partnering with the couple to form a marriage, which is a new link in the chain of their families. The partnership itself is premised on a shared virtuous vision that is greater than themselves. Ask yourselves, "What is so important in life that each of us would commit to, and what is so meaningful that our children and future generations would also commit?"

Covenants

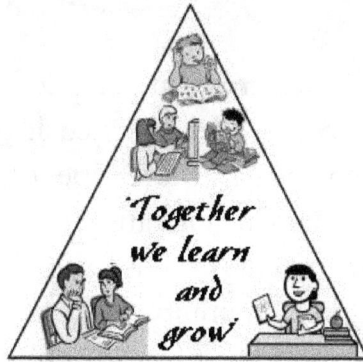

"Covenant" is a good word because as a reciprocal agreement it has higher-level ethical, religious, and spiritual connotations.

While you cannot fully foresee the road ahead, as in many worthy life challenges, have faith that you will find your way. With research, reflection and dialogue we can bridge the gap between what we know and do not know, and learn how to apply what we know.

Combined efforts to craft a shared vision and guiding principles require patience, respect, and asking good questions. Families are challenged to learn together.

If creative transformation is not a part of a family's commitments, then resignation is the likely default, and a couple will not meet the challenges of today or tomorrow. Resignation encourages acceptance of things undesirable and can even sow the seeds of cynicism and alienation in the next generations.

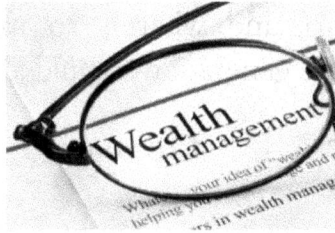

From a wealth preservation perspective, creating Family Covenants can be a sound practice in risk management. Arguably, in many ways, the scope of life challenges is greater for the Millennial generation and Generation Z than it was for their parents. Thus, the younger generation requires more skill, humility, and support from their parents and family. They could choose to be merely independent and assert the naive authenticity of *doing their own thing* while their parents stand on the sidelines hoping and praying for the best; or they could wisely choose to be interdependent with their parents and parents-in-law.

Crafting the Covenants

Many Western couples, depending upon their religious tradition, craft vows of commitment. In *A Better Way To Marry*, not only do the two candidates create their "Engaged Couple Covenants," parents are also encouraged to concurrently craft their "Parents' Covenants." The Engaged Couple and Parents' Covenants are essentially shared vision and commitment statements and guiding principles, which can be developed over a period of several weeks through e-mails, phone calls, or personal visits. The process of creating a covenant can facilitate mutual learning about one's similarities and different points of view and styles of collaboration.

Joint Inter-Family Covenant

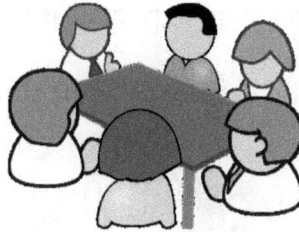

There is another covenant that can be created as part of the Engagement Commitment Ceremony. It is a joint "Inter-Family Covenant." From the perspective of a society, marriage is the means through which a community of people perpetuates itself. Marriage creates kinship and various obligations.

To minimize surprises and strengthen a foundation of interdependence, the engaged couple and their parents collectively discuss and express in terms of vision and principles what they would agree to do as families. It can be a challenge to do that; however, the greater challenge is to live up to our fondest ideals.

Pre-Marriage Preparation
Planning to Become "As One": Sexuality

The period between the engagement ceremony and the wedding is an opportunity for couples to demonstrate their lifelong commitments by maintaining sexual self-discipline and restraint until they are married. Humans are endowed with reason, will, spiritual intelligence and a conscience to regulate their appetites for healthy purposes. An engaged couple best clarify their sexual expectations by reviewing, and correcting as needed, their knowledge levels of the male and female anatomies, and about initiating sexual relations when beginning married life. Sexuality is widely obscured with unrealistic expectations.

Slower is Better

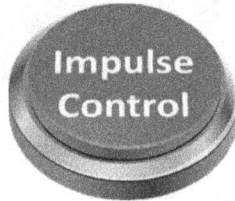

For example, unprepared young males are inclined to be impulsive when initiating sexual relations with their brides and may fail to realize that they can physically and emotionally injure them if they do not act slowly, knowledgably, and with thoughtful sensitivity. Experiences during the first intimate moments of marriage can leave long-lasting memories.

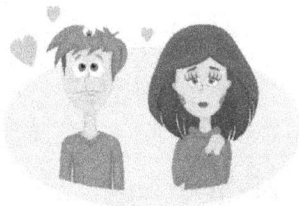

Alternatively, there are young men who have performance anxiety when they begin married life. They may worry that condoms will impair their ability to perform. Expressing such fears honestly can help manage them. Worrying about performing and *doing it right* can distract from emotional and spiritual connection and intimacy, which is at the heart of sexuality.

Although women may feel ready to have sexual relations, they may not have orgasms at first. When the Hollywood expectations of mutual orgasms fail to occur, a young couple may become disillusioned and lament, "Is that all there is?"

When a married couple become physically intimate, they may need more time to snuggle and physically transition through layers of physical and emotional sensitivity.

There are many myths related to sexuality that may influence the expectations of a young couple when they first become romantically involved.

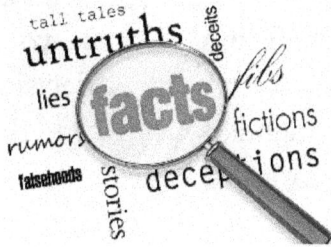

Consider the myth that an unbroken hymen is a sign of virginity. Actually, it can break due to exercise, inserting a tampon, or other reasons. In certain cultures, a broken hymen separated from the vaginal walls can lead to the presumption of premarital sexual intercourse and subject a woman to public humiliation or worse.

Parents may have difficulty or reluctance speaking with their children about sex because they are embarrassed to do so or they do not know how to talk about it.

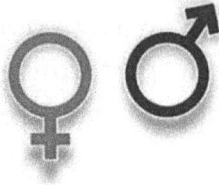

If parents do not teach their children about sex, they may be the only ones who do not. Sex talk is everywhere in our sex-obsessed society. It is discussed on TV, in the movies, the Internet, at school, and by their friends. Children and adults commonly get sexual information from unreliable and misleading sources.

Choosing a Contraceptive

In preparation for an approaching marriage or during marriage, if a couple considers birth control, they best discuss its risks, benefits, and be clear who is assuming which risks and who is benefitting. Often young women make their birth control decisions based on recommendations from their friends. Reading stories or hearing that the risks of female birth control are minimal can be interpreted as "it's okay."

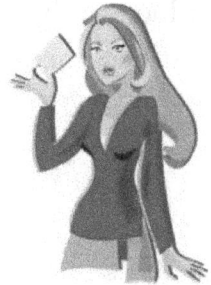

It is important to be aware of the known risks associated with each contraceptive choice. These risks include but are not limited to blood clots, stroke, aggravated high blood pressure, heart, liver and gallbladder disease. If a woman does not closely monitor the creeping side effects of contraceptive hormones, a blood clot can move from her calf to her thigh to her lung and elsewhere and become life threatening; ulcers can also form in the uterus and infertility can result.[123]

Risk is Risk

It is easy for a man to gladly acquiesce to his fiancée who volunteers to use the patch, ring or the pill during marriage. However, the risks are real and side effects are more common than most realize. Women often assume the negative consequences of birth control. It is important to consistently monitor side effects and to re-evaluate the effectiveness of birth control and each partner's satisfaction with a particular choice of contraception.

Women may confer with gynecologists who can explain birth control alternatives and their risks. However, risk is risk and the jury is still out regarding the long-term consequences of contraceptives, and you may be among the few who suffer from the side effects.

When a couple engages to be married, they form a partnership and should thoughtfully plan for the future and consider the highest well-being of one another. They are to become "as one." If you are a man, treat the body of your spouse with as much or more care as you do your own. If couples decide that female contraceptives are too risky, then the future husband may decide that he does not want his future wife exposed to them. He and she may decide that he use condoms. Assure that birth control is a thoughtful, informed, and mutual decision.

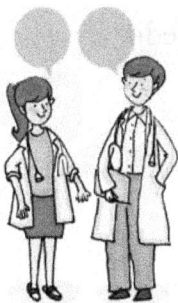

Doctors may be able to explain the human anatomy and the medical aspects of sexuality; however, they are not always the best persons to explain how to make sex more pleasurable and meaningful.

Doctors have their own preconceived notions about sexuality, intimacy, and what a man and woman are and should be able to do. In certain circumstances those notions can compromise the trust between couples. For instance, a young woman informed her male gynecologist that both she and her husband had been abstinent before their forthcoming marriage. The doctor casually asserted that he did not believe it and that no man could or should abstain, which implied that she and her fiancé were dishonest. Imagine if you were that woman.

An engaged couple is a partnership. They will learn together. Learning with your partner while sharing lifelong commitments is liberating. It encourages the honesty and vulnerability necessary for true intimacy to develop.

The engagement period is an opportunity for a couple to expand their capacities for trust, which serve as pathways for enhanced intimacy. Some women and men are not emotionally ready to initiate sexual relations in marriage. If so, are they ready to be married?

Your Story

If you will be planning your wedding, your preparations will be part of the story that others will ask about once they learn that you are engaged. Many will immediately want to know how the "big question was asked," and when and where the big wedding will be held so they can plan to attend. The pressure to conform to their expectations will escalate.

Surprise them with the story of how you and your spouse-to-be genuinely assured yourselves that you were ready for marriage through your reflective journey of self-discovery and mutual discovery, exchanging your autobiographies and biographies, interviews, heartfelt discussions with your spouse-to-be, and with your parents and in-laws-to-be.

You will need some space and time to plan for the wedding. Your friends will want to give advice, especially the ones recently married. Graciously thank them for their advice. As in other things, take the best and leave the rest.

Being ready for marriage precedes preparing for the wedding. Your time and investment assure that you, your future spouse and both of your parents are prepared to travel life together.

Our hope is that *A Better Way To Marry* can contribute to elevating the position of parents and empower them to be wisdom givers for marriage. We also hope that the insights provided here will enable single adults to marry wisely and marry well.

ABOUT THE AUTHORS

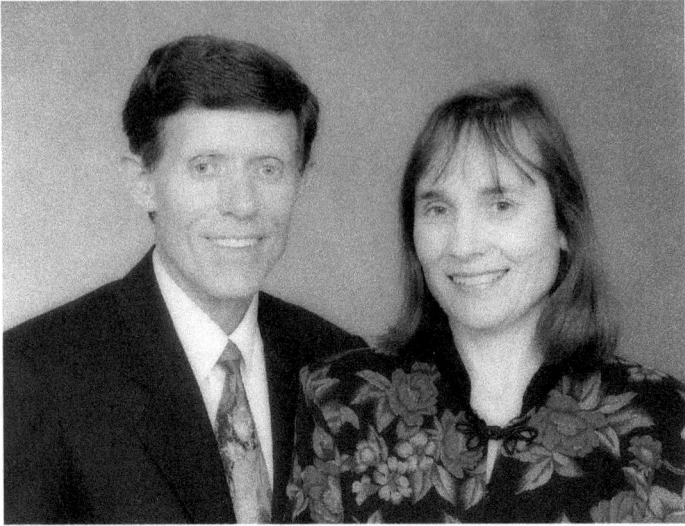

Ken and Verena Hardman, married for more than 35 years, are parents to three daughters, two of whom are happily married through *A Better Way To Marry* process, a son, and two grandchildren. Ken is a real estate broker by profession, and Verena is a mother by vocation. They have partnered to initiate and support family and community-based projects that have focused on marriage, parent-child and family development, intercultural and interreligious cooperation. Their projects have ranged from co-producing and directing *Toward Intercultural Understanding*, a local cable television program, managing educational programs for middle school and high school students promoting altruism and strengthening parent-child-teacher relationships, conducting in-home marriage enrichment seminars, to supporting local programs addressing homelessness, refugee and immigrant resettlement.

They have also edited *Through Afghan Eyes: Survival during the Soviet-Afghan War and Warnings to the West Before 9/11*, the memoir of their long-time friend and colleague, Sher Ahmad.

Ken is a Vietnam veteran. Verena shares his special concerns for those that have served and are currently serving in the military. There are common denominators between the military and refugee/immigrant communities. They include that their marriages and families face extra challenges and are experiencing rising numbers of divorces. Ken and Verena hope that *A Better Way To Marry* will well serve those communities and others.

ENDNOTES

Preface Notes

[1] Joseph Campbell, *The Power of Myth with Bill Moyers,* Betty Sue Flowers, ed., (New York: Anchor Books, 1991), Chapter I.

[2] K.A. Bogle, "The Shift from Dating to Hooking up in College: What Scholars Have Missed." *Sociology Compass,* (2007), 775-788. doi:10.1111/j.1751-9020.2007.00031.x.

[3] "National Intimate Partner and Sexual Violence Survey: An Overview of 2010 Summary Report Findings." *www.cdc.gov,* https://www.cdc.gov/violenceprevention/pdf/nisvs_report2010-a.pdf, and

"Understanding Teen Dating Violence." *www.cdc.gov.* www.cdc.gov/ViolencePrevention/pdf/TeenDatingViolence2012-a.pdf. "Dating violence is a type of intimate partner violence. It occurs between two people in a close relationship. The nature of dating violence can be physical, emotional, or sexual."

[4] Alexandra Brodsky, "'Rape-adjacent': Imagining Legal Responses to Nonconsensual Condom Removal," *Columbia Journal of Gender and Law, Vol. 32, No. 2, 2017,* https://cjgl.journals.cdrs.columbia.edu/wp-content/uploads/sites/18/2017/04/Brodsky_Final_PRINT.pdf.

Robert Glatter, M.D., "'Stealthing': The Disturbing New Sex Trend You Need To Know About," *Forbes,* April 29, 2017, https://www.forbes.com/sites/robertglatter/2017/04/29/stealthing-the-disturbing-new-sex-trend-you-need-to-know-about/#5ca3d20f1b07 .

[5] Greg Hodge, "The Ugly Truth of Online Dating: Top 10 Lies Told by Internet Daters," *http://www.huffingtonpost.com* , December 10, 2012, https://www.huffingtonpost.com/greg-hodge/online-dating-lies_b_1930053.html .

[6] John M. Gottman, and Nan Silver, *The Seven Principles For Making Marriage Work* (New York: Three Rivers Press, 1999), 27-34. Gottman calls these behaviors the four horsemen.

[7] Jeffrey A. Lieberman, M.D., *Shrinks: The Untold Story of Psychiatry,* (New York: Brown and Company, 2015), 48. Lieberman is a psychiatrist and former president of the American Psychiatric Association (APA). He provides an informative historical review of the psychiatric profession who states "Freud ended up leading psychiatry in an intellectual desert for more than a half-century."

[8] Ibid.

[9] Gottman, *The Seven Principles For Making Marriage Work*, Chapter 1.

[10] "Young, Underemployed and Optimistic: Coming of Age, Slowly, in a Tough Economy", *Pew Research Center*, February 9, 2012, Ch. 1: Overview, http://www.pewsocialtrends.org/2012/02/09/young-underemployed-and-optimistic/2/#chapter-1-overview.Pew Research Center 2012.

[11] Ron Lieber, "From Parents, a Living Inheritance", *www.nytimes.com*, September 21, 2012, http://www.nytimes.com/2012/09/22/your-money/the-hidden-inheritance-many-parents-already-provide.html?pagewanted=all. Also, AARP compared the responses of young adults today ages 21 through 26 with those of Boomers in their early twenties regarding their parental relationships when they were in their early 20s. When Boomers were young, 32% lived with their parents. Today 43% live with their parents. From the "AARP Generations Study", *AARP*, December 2012/January2013, 55.

Chapter 1 Notes

[12] Distinctions between the generations are made in various ways such as the Lost Generation (those who came of age during WWI), the Greatest Generation (those who were young adults in the WWII era), the Silent Generation (children during WWII and young adults during Korean War), the Baby Boomers, Generation X, Generation Y, and Generation Z. Each generation has its own set of traits and cultural impact.

[13] James E. Hughes, Jr., Esq., *Family Wealth: Keeping It in the Family--How Family Members and Their Advisors Preserve Human, Intellectual, and Financial Assets for Generations* (New York: Bloomberg Press, 2004), 13-14.

[14] Ibid.

[15] Richard A. Morris and Jayne A. Pearl, *Kids, Wealth, and Consequences: Ensuring a Responsible Financial Future for the Next Generation* (Hoboken, New Jersey: John Wiley & Sons, Inc., 2010), 2.

[16] George Lakoff, *Moral Politics: What Conservatives Know That Liberals Don't* (Chicago: The University of Chicago Press, 1996), 36.

Chapter 2 Notes

[17] Martin E.P. Seligman, *Flourish: A Visionary New Understanding of Happiness and Well-Being* (New York: Free Press, 2011), 60.

[18] Ibid., 59.

[19] Thomas Lewis, M.D., Fari Amini, M.D., and Richard Lannon, M.D., *A General Theory of Love* (New York: Vintage Books, 2000), 8-10, 102-103. In 1990, George Franklin had been convicted of killing an eight-year-old girl, 20 years earlier. It was based on his daughter suddenly remembering seeing him do it. There were no witnesses, no physical evidence, no DNA. A

psychiatrist testified that the daughter's memory was indisputably recovered forgotten memory. The jury believed them. After five years a federal court threw out the conviction. Franklin's daughter had "remembered" two other murders committed by her father which he could not have committed.

[20] Ibid.

[21] Lloyd Sederer, "Overprescribing and Underperforming: Mental health care for youth in the U.S. relies too heavily on antipsychotics and too little on comprehensive treatment," *www.usnews.com*, July 2, 2015, www.usnews.com/opinion/blogs/policy-dose/2015/07/02/the-us-is-overprescribing-antipsychotic-medications-to-youth.

[22] George E.Vaillant, *Aging Well* (Boston: Little, Brown and Company, 2002).

[23] Ibid., 40-41.

[24] Seligman, *Flourish*, 157-158.

[25] Young monkeys were offered a choice between two surrogate mothers: a wire mesh container with a milk feeding bottle and a terrycloth object that resembled a monkey—it offered no milk. After the monkeys acquired the milk from the wire mesh mother, they went to the terry cloth mother.

[26] David Brooks, *The Social Animal: The Hidden Sources of Love, Character, and Achievement* (New York: Random House, 2011), xv.

[27] Dorothy Tennov, *Love and Limerence: The Experience of Being in Love* (New York: Scarborough House, 1999), 15, 171.

[28] Helen Fisher, Ph.D., *Why We Love: The Nature And Chemistry of Romantic Love* (New York: Henry Holt And Company, 2004), xiv, 72. 182. See also Alice Park, "Forget Pain Pills, Fall in Love Instead." *Time.com*, October 14, 2010, http://healthland.time.com/2010/10/14/forget-pain-pills-fall-in-love-instead/. Park reports the pain management research of Stanford University professor Dr. Sean Mackey in which functional MRI (fMRI) scans suggest that the falling in love and in love experience are similar to addictive drugs like cocaine that can dull pain perception.

[29] Professor Jason M. Satterfield, *Cognitive Behavioral Therapy: Techniques for Retraining Your Brain, Course Guidebook* (Chantilly, Virginia: The Teaching Company, 2015), 4. John Hopkins Medicine Health Library's "Mental Health Disorder Statistics" reports 26% of Americans 18 years and older suffer from a diagnosable mental disorder in a given year like depression, anxiety disorder, OCD, PTSD, phobias, https://www.hopkinsmedicine.org/healthlibrary/conditions/mental_health _disorders/mental_health_disorder_statistics_85,P00753. A May 15, 2015 blog post by Thomas Insel at the National Institute of Mental Health

estimates that the number is 1 in 5 adult Americans (about 43 million) who had a diagnosable mental disorder within the past year: https://www.nimh.nih.gov/about/directors/thomas-insel/blog/2015/mental-health-awareness-month-by-the-numbers.shtml.
³⁰ "Mental Health By The Numbers," *National Alliance on Mental Illness (NAMI)*, https://www.nami.org/Learn-More/Mental-Health-By-the-Numbers. The 60% statistic within this report came from http://www.samhsa.gov/data/sites/default/files/NSDUH-FRR1-2014/NSDUH-FRR1-2014.pdf.
³¹ Deidre McPhillips, "U.S. Among Most Depressed Countries in the World," *www.usnews.com*, September 14, 2016, https://www.usnews.com/news/best-countries/articles/2016-09-14/the-10-most-depressed-countries.
³² Ibid., xiv-xv.

³³ Seligman, Flourish, 45-46. Seligman laments how three separate times his proposals to the National Institute of Mental Health (NIMH) were rejected and unreviewed. They were to fund "[breakthrough] positive psychology exercises on the web—that is dirt cheap, massively disseminated, and at least as effective as therapy and drugs." "The first dirty little secret of biological psychiatry and of clinical psychology is that they both have given up the notion of cure. Cure takes too long if it can be done at all, and only brief treatment is reimbursed by insurance companies. So therapy and drugs are now entirely about short-term crisis management and about dispensing cosmetic treatments."

The World Health Organization (WHO) reported in 2017 that depression is the leading worldwide cause of ill health and disability. It has globally increased 18% between 2005 to 2015 to affect 300 million people.
³⁴ Bella DePaulo Ph.D., "What Is the Divorce Rate, Really?", www.psychologytoday.com, February 2, 2017, https://www.psychologytoday.com/blog/living-single/201702/what-is-the-divorce-rate-really. This article examines the opinions of family scholar Paul Amato, Claire Cain Miller, Steven Ruggles, and Justin Wolfers who debate whether about 50% of marriages end in divorce.
³⁵ Beck Institute for Cognitive Behavior Therapy, https://beckinstitute.org/cognitive-model/.
³⁶ Stephen R. Covey, *The 8th Habit: From Effectiveness to Greatness* (New York: Free Press, 2004), 65.

³⁷ Ibid., 53-54.

³⁸ Seligman, *Flourish*, 150.

³⁹ Ibid., 127-128, 144.

⁴⁰ P.D. Harms, Mitchel N. Herian, Dina V. Krasikova, Adam Vanhove, Paul B. Lester, "The Comprehensive Soldier Fitness Program Evaluation. Report #4: Evaluation of Master Resilience Training and Mental and Behavioral Health Outcomes," University of Nebraska-Lincoln, April 2013, http://digitalcommons.unl.edu/cgi/viewcontent.cgi?article=1009&context=pdharms.

⁴¹ Brad Broker, "U.S. Soldiers Have Mental Health Disorders Prior to Enlisting," *www.physiciansnews.com*, March 4, 2014, http://www.physiciansnews.com/2014/03/04/u-s-soldiers-have-mental-health-disorders-prior-to-enlisting. While some early studies have surmised that the program has not been effective to prevent suicides, the Army cites data that in 2013 improvements were materializing and there was about a 20% decrease in suicides. Suicides and PTSD are complex problems difficult to measure, especially when many soldiers were mentally ill before enlisting. The recent *Army Study to Assess Risk and Resilience in Servicemembers* (Army STARRS) reported that almost 50% of soldiers who had attempted suicide had done so before entering the Army. Somehow, they got through the initial enlistment screening process. Usually military applicants who disclose a history of suicide attempts are excluded from service. Also 75% of soldiers who exhibited signs of anger disorder had evidenced it before enlisting. The military seeks to do a better job of screening applicants.

⁴² Seligman, *Flourish*, 150.

⁴³ Thomas L. Friedman, *Thank You for Being Late: An Optimist's Guide To Thriving In The Age Of Accelerations* (New York: Farrar, Straus and Giroux, 2016), 68.

⁴⁴ American Academy of Family Physicians (AAFP), "Violence (Position Paper)," www.aafp.org, 2014, http://www.aafp.org/about/policies/all/violence.html.

⁴⁵ "The National Intimate Partner and Sexual Violence Survey: 2010 Summary Report, Executive Summary," *Centers for Disease Control and Prevention: National Center for Injury Prevention and Control*, November 2011, https://www.cdc.gov/violenceprevention/pdf/nisvs_report2010-a.pdf.

⁴⁶ Peter Senge, *The Fifth Discipline: The Art & Practice of The Learning Organization* (New York: Doubleday, 1990), 142.

Chapter 3 Notes

⁴⁷ Paul R. Amato, Alan Booth, David R. Johnson, and Stacy J. Rogers, *Alone Together* (Cambridge, Massachusetts: Harvard University Press, 2007), 251.

⁴⁸ Ibid., 255.

[49] Mueller, P. S., Plevak, D. J., & Rummans, T. A. (2001). Religious involvement, spirituality, and medicine: Implications for clinical practice. Mayo Clinic Proceedings, 76(12), 1225-1235; http://www.mayoclinicproceedings.org/article/S0025-6196(11)62799-7/fulltext;

[50] Peter Senge, *The Fifth Discipline*, 142.

[51] Although spirituality and religion converge in many ways, since many people negatively react to the word *spirituality* thinking it is about religion, it's helpful to distinguish it from the word *religion*. The Army and holistic physicians do so. The Army affirms that its "Spiritual Fitness Module" is not theologically based. Rather it is premised on living by a code that serves a purpose(s) greater than the self. A person's spiritual core is formed over time through a variety of sources: philosophical, cultural, religious and psychological teachings, and life experiences. See Seligman, *Flourish*, 149-151. The word "religion" tends to be viewed as membership in an institution with rituals and traditions and doctrines.

[52] Senge, *The Fifth Discipline*, 142.

[53] Mark Dummett, 'Not so happily ever after as Indian divorce rate doubles," *BBC News, South Asia*, January 1, 2011, http://www.bbc.com/news/world-south-asia-12094360.

[54] Martin Rossman, M.D., *The Worry Solution: Using Your Healing Mind to Turn Stress and Anxiety into Confidence and Happiness*. (New York: Crown Archetype, 2010), xiii.

[55] Rossman, *The Worry Solution*, 17.

[56] Ibid. Also, *Facts & Statistics*, Anxiety And Depression Association Of America, https://adaa.org/about-adaa/press-room/facts-statistics, Updated August, 2017.

[57] "Military Divorce Risk Increases With Lengthy Deployments," *www.huffingtonpost.com*, September 3, 2013, http://www.huffingtonpost.com/2013/09/03/military-divorce_n_3861441.html.

[58] Roy F. Baumeister and John Tierney, *Willpower: Rediscovering the Greatest Human Strength* (New York: Penguin Books, 2011), 1.

[59] Don Emerson Davis, Jr., and Joshua N. Hook, "Measuring Humility and Its Positive Effects," *Association for Psychological Science*, October 2013, https://www.psychologicalscience.org/observer/measuring-humility-and-its-positive-effects#.WWBkhojyuUk.

[60] Ibid.

61 Science Daily, "Abuse, lack of parental warmth in childhood linked to multiple health risks in adulthood," *www.sciencedaily.com*. September 26, 2013, www.sciencedaily.com/releases/2013/09/130926205005.htm.

62 Seligman, *Flourish*, 189.

Chapter 4 Notes

63 Eric W.Corty, PhD, Jenay M. Guardiani, BS,"Canadian And American Sex Therapists' Perceptions Of Normal And Abnormal Ejaculatory Latencies: How Long Should Intercourse Last?", *The Journal of Sexual Medicine: An Official Journal of The International Society for Sexual Medicine*, May 2005, Vol. 5, Issue 5, Pages 1251-1256, http://www.jsm.jsexmed.org/article/S1743-6095(15)32017-8/fulltext. "Too short" a time was 1 to 2 minutes and "too long" was 10 to 30 minutes. These results were speculated to possibly "be beneficial to couples in treatment for sexual problems by normalizing expectations."

64 Shmuley Boteach, Rabbi, *The Kosher Sutra: 8 Sacred Secrets for Reigniting Desire and Restoring Passion for Life* (New York: Harper-Collins Publishers, 2009), 34, 37, 52, 53.

65 Ibid., 52-102.

66 Janet M. Ruane and Karen A. Cerulo, *Second Thoughts: Sociology Challenges Conventional Wisdom* (Los Angeles: Sage, 2015), 191.

67 The rise of chronic loneliness during the past 20 years was reported in the research of John Cacioppo, Director of the Center for Cognitive and Social Neuroscience at the University of Chicago. He explained its dangers in an interview with Laura Entis, "Chronic Loneliness Is a Modern-Day Epidemic," *www.fortune.com*, June 22, 2016, http://fortune.com/2016/06/22/loneliness-is-a-modern-day-epidemic/ .

68 Merrit Kennedy, "U.K. Now Has A Minister For Loneliness," NPR, January 17, 2018, https://www.npr.org/sections/thetwo-way/2018/01/17/578645954/u-k-now-has-a-minister-for-loneliness.

69 Caroline Beaton explains two reasons why loneliness is most prevalent among Millennials in "Why Millennials Are Lonely," www.forbes.com, February 9, 2017, https://www.forbes.com/sites/carolinebeaton/2017/02/09/why-millennials-are-lonely/#53c6204c7c35. Loneliness is contagious and "the Internet makes it viral."

70 Susan Pinker, *The Village Effect: How Face-to-Fact Contact Can Make Us Healthier and Happier* (Toronto: Random House Canada, 2014), 9.

71 Miller McPherson, Lynn Smith-Lovin, Matthew E. Brashears, "Social Isolation in America: Changes in Core Discussion Networks over Two Decades," *American Sociological Review*, Volume 71, Issue 3, June 1, 2006,

353-375,
http://journals.sagepub.com/doi/abs/10.1177/000312240607100301.
[72] Guy Winch, Ph.D. "10 Surprising Facts About Loneliness,"
www.psychologytoday.com, October 14, 2014,
https://www.psychologytoday.com/blog/the-squeaky-wheel/201410/10-surprising-facts-about-loneliness.
[73] This US Census Bureau data is reported by Courtney Coren, "Census
Bureau: More Americans Marrying Twice or More," *www.newsmax.com*,
March 16, 2015, https://www.newsmax.com/us/marriage-census-bureau-divorced-adults/2015/03/16/id/630369/.
[74] Susan Brown and I-Fen Lin, "The Gray Divorce Revolution: Rising
Divorce Among Middle-aged and Older Adults, 1990-2009," *The Journals of
Gerontology: Series B 67 (6): 731-741,* November 11, 2012,
https://www.ncbi.nlm.nih.gov/pmc/articles/PMC3478728/,
https://www.ncbi.nlm.nih.gov/pubmed/23052366.
[75] Tom W. Smith, "American Sexual Behavior: Trends, Socio-Demographic
Difference, and Risk Behavior," GSS Topical Report No. 25 (Chicago:
National Opinion Research Center, University of Chicago 2006, March
2006), 12-14.
http://www.norc.org/PDFs/Publications/AmericanSexualBehavior2006.pdf .
[76] Milton Lakin, MD, "Erectile Dysfunction," *Cleveland Clinic Center for
Continuing Education*, November 2012 ,
http://www.clevelandclinicmeded.com/medicalpubs/diseasemanagement/endocrinology/erectile-dysfunction/. Erectile dysfunction is defined as "the
inability to develop and maintain an erection for satisfactory sexual
intercourse or activity in the absence of an ejaculatory disorder such as
premature ejaculation…. There is no universally agreed criteria for how
consistent the problem has to be and for what duration has to be and for
what duration it needs to be present to fulfill the definition. A period of
persistence of longer than 3 months has been suggested as a reasonable
clinical guideline." "Experience of sexual dysfunction was more likely
among men in poor physical and emotional health. It was also concluded
that sexual dysfunction is an important public health concern and added
that emotional issues are likely to contribute to the experience of these
problems."
[77] Denis de Rougemont, *Love in the Western World*, (New Jersey: Princeton
University Press,1983), 16, 17. "Novels and plays subsist on the so-called
'breakdown of marriage'. Probably, also they help to prolong the
breakdown, on the one hand by extolling what religion regards as a crime
and law as an infringement, and, on the other hand, by making fun of this

and drawing from it an inexhaustible fund of situations either comic or shameless."

[78] "The Impact of Pornography on Children," *American College of Pediatricians*, June, 2016, https://www.acpeds.org/the-college-speaks/position-statements/the-impact-of-pornography-on-children. This survey referenced a 2008 article in the *Journal of Adolescent Research* which revealed that 67% of young men and 49% of young women found pornography acceptable.

[79] Ibid.

[80] Ibid.

[81] Lauren Dubinsky, "What I Wish I'd Known Before Watching Porn," *www.huffingtonpost.com,* September 22, 2012, http://www.huffingtonpost.com/lauren-dubinsky/porn-addiction_b_1686481.html.

[82] "Attitudes about sexuality and aging," Harvard health Publishing: Harvard Medical School, March 17, 2017, https://www.health.harvard.edu/staying-healthy/attitudes-about-sexuality-and-aging.

[83] Ibid.

[84] Covey, *The 8th Habit*, 65.

[85] G.P. Putnam's Sons, *The Oxford American College Dictionary*, 443.

[86] See Rabbi Shmuley Boteach, *Kosher Sex: A Recipe for Passion and Intimacy* (London: Duckworth Overlook, 1998) and Rabbi Shmuley Boteach, *The Kosher Sutra.*

[87] Gottman, *The Seven Principles For Making Marriage Work*, 4.

[88] "What Is Forgiveness?", *Greater Good Magazine*, The Greater Good Science Center at the University of California, Berkeley, https://greatergood.berkeley.edu/forgiveness/definition.

[89] Elizabeth Gilbert, *Big Magic* (San Francisco: Thorndike Press, 2015), 224-231.

[90] Galen Guengerich, Ph.D., 2014. "Why Creativity Is Risky Business: The perils posed by creativity aren't the obvious ones," *www.psychologytoday.com,* February 27, 2014, https://www.psychologytoday.com/blog/the-search-meaning/201402/why-creativity-is-risky-business.

Chapter 5 Notes

[91] Gottman, *The Seven Principles For Making Marriage Work*, 13-14.

[92] Justin A. Lavner and Thomas N. Bradbury, "Why Do Even Satisfied Newlyweds Eventually Go on to Divorce?," *Journal of Family Psychology* 26 (1): 1-10, September 14, 2011,

---

http://marriage.psych.ucla.edu/publications/Lavner%20%26%20Bradbury%202012.pdf?attredirects=0.

[93] Gottman, *The Seven Principles For Making Marriage Work*, 27-34.

[94] Ibid., 13.

[95] Covey, *The 8th Habit*, 151. "Interdependency is an awareness of the reality that all of life is connected, particularly with organizations and complementary teams that are attempting to win and keep the loyalty of customers, associates, suppliers and owners. Independent thinking in an interdependent reality would again be analogous to playing tennis with a golf club or thinking analog ideas in a digital world."

[96] Stephen R. Covey, *The 3d Alternative: Solving Life's Most Difficult Problems* (New York: Free Press, 2011), 41.

[97] Stephen R. Covey, *The 7 Habits of Highly Effective Families* (New York: Golden Books, 1997), 179.

[98] Michael Dues, *The Art of Conflict Management: Achieving Solutions for Life, Work, and Beyond* (Chantilly, Virginia: The Teaching Company, 2010), 10-11.

[99] Senge, *The Fifth Discipline*, 170, 171.

[100] Josh Levs, *All In: How Our Work-First Culture Fails Dads, Families, and Businesses--And How We Can Fix It Together* (New York: Harper Collins Publishers, 2015).

[101] His were four temperaments: melancholic, phlegmatic, choleric and sanguine.

[102] The Myers-Briggs Type Indicator (MBTI) personality questionnaire was created by a mother (Katherine Cook Briggs) and daughter (Isabel Briggs Myers) team who were inspired by Carl Jung's theory of psychological types. See http://www.myersbriggs.org/my-mbti-personality-type/mbti-basics/.

[103] Peter Urs Bender, http://www.peterursbender.com/quiz/.

[104] The Flag Page, http://www.flagpage.com/.

[105] Diane H. Felmlee, "Fatal Attractions: Affection and Disaffection in Intimate Relationships," *Journal of Social and Personal Relationships* 12 (2), (1995), 295-312, http://journals.sagepub.com/doi/abs/10.1177/0265407595122009.

[106] Ayala Malach Pines, *Falling in Love: Why We Choose the Lovers We Choose* (New York: Taylor & Francis Group, 2005), 184.

Chapter 6 Notes

[107] Aaron Smith and Monica Anderson, "5 facts about online dating," *www.pewresearch.org,* February 29, 2016, http://www.pewresearch.org/fact-tank/2016/02/29/5-facts-about-online-dating/.

[108] W. Bradford Wilcox and Elizabeth Marquardt, eds., *The State of Our Unions. Marriage in America 2010: When Marriage Disappears: The New Middle America* (Charlottesville, VA: National Marriage Project and the Institute for American Values, 2010), 23-24, http://nationalmarriageproject.org/wp-content/uploads/2012/06/Union_11_12_10.pdf.

[109] Amber and David Lapp, "Looking for Marriage in Middle America," *Institute For American Values,* April 2013: 4, http://americanvalues.org/catalog/pdfs/2013-04.pdf.

[110] Aziz Ansari and Eric Klinenberg, *Modern Romance* (New York: Penguin Press, 2015), 42.

Chapter 7 Notes

[111] Greg Hodge, "The Ugly Truth of Online Dating: Top 10 Lies Told by Internet Daters," *http://www.huffingtonpost.com ,* December 10, 2012, https://www.huffingtonpost.com/greg-hodge/online-dating-lies_b_1930053.html .

[112] "Of Love and Scams: How to Tell if You're Being Catfished," *www.org,* May 18, 2016, https://www.bbb.org/sacramento/news-events/consumer-tips/2016/05/of-love-and-scams-how-to-tell-if-youre-being-catfished/.

Chapter 8 Notes

[113] Helen Branswell, "Gonorrhea May Soon Be Resistant to all Antibiotics," *www.scientificamerican.com,* July 15, 2016, http://www.scientificamerican.com/article/gonorrhea-may-soon-be-resistant-to-all-antibiotics/. More than 350,000 people were diagnosed with gonorrhea in 2014.

[114] John Van Epp, Ph.D., *How To Avoid Falling in Love With a Jerk* (New York, et.al.: McGraw Hill, 2007), 78.

[115] Lori Gottlieb, *Marry Him: The Case for Settling for Mr. Good Enough* (New York: Penguin Group, 2010). See also her March 2008 article in *the Atlantic* which launched her 2010 book, https://www.theatlantic.com/magazine/archive/2008/03/marry-him/306651/.

[116] As a real estate broker, Ken used the method to negotiate real estate contracts, and to mediate landlord/tenant rental disputes with a very high success rate. We have also used it during our marriage and for family projects. It can be part of the courtship process.

[117] He has gleaned from those studies and produced *The Seven Principles For Making Marriage Work*. Similarly, Stephen Covey refers to exemplary marriages within *The 7 Habits of Highly Effective Families*. We learned from them and many other sources of research and experience. With over 35 years of marriage we recognized their value.

[118] Lewis, *A General Theory of Love*, 12-13.

Chapter 9 Notes

[119] Annie Lowrey, "The Great Recession Is Still With Us: The downturn left the country poorer and more unequal than it would have been otherwise," December 1, 2017, https://www.theatlantic.com/business/archive/2017/12/great-recession-still-with-us/547268/.

[120] Bruce Drake, "6 new findings about Millennials," Pew Research Center, March 7, 2014, http://www.pewresearch.org/fact-tank/2014/03/07/6-new-findings-about-millennials/.

[121] Attributed to "The Constitution of the Iroquois Nations: The Great Binding Law," http://en.wikipedia.org/wiki/Seven_generation_sustainability. It appears that the language of "seventh generation" did not come from that specific document, though. Nevertheless, it does include generation-thinking language: "Look and listen for the welfare of the whole people and have always in view not only the present but also the coming generations,…"

[122] James E. Hughes, Jr., Esq., "A Reflection on the Role of Elders in a System of Family Governance." *James E. Hughes, Jr.*, 2002, www.jameshughes.com/articles/Elders.pdf, and "A Reflection On The Role of Aunts And Uncles In A System Of Family Governance."

[123] The Mayo Clinic Staff, "Dep-Provera (contraceptive injection): Risks," December 14, 2014, http://www.mayoclinic.org/tests-procedures/depo-provera/basics/risks/prc-20013801. Among the list of side effects of Depo-Provera contraceptive injections are potential loss of bone mineral density, delay in return to fertility, acne, breast sores, decreased interest in sex, headaches, weight gain, depression and more.

Chana Gazit, *The Pill*, Documentary Film, Directed by Chana Gazit and David Steward/, (2003: WGBH, PBS, 2003). The 2003 documentary may seem dated; however, it provides an interesting historical overview of the birth control pill and its risks which are not dated.

PlannedParenthood.org warns that "[l]ike with all medications, the pill isn't for everyone…. If you're over 35 and a smoker, you shouldn't use the pill or any other kind of birth control that contains the hormone estrogen." It provides other warnings: https://www.plannedparenthood.org/learn/birth-control/birth-control-pill/how-safe-is-the-birth-control-pill.

www.ingramcontent.com/pod-product-compliance
Lightning Source LLC
Chambersburg PA
CBHW050111280326
41933CB00010B/1051